Going Back To The Basics of Human Health

Avoiding the Fads, the Trends, and the Bold-faced Lies

Revised Edition

MARY FROST, M.A.

Frost, Mary
Going Back To The Basics of Human Health
Avoiding The Fads, The Trends, and The Bold-Faced
Lies/Mary Frost

ISBN 0-9656940-8-9
1. Health and Fitness

Manufactured in the United States of America

First Edition, February 1997

Cover art by Joel Sharp

To Dr. Royal Lee, who was and still is a beacon of light for all of us who want to be healthy.

To my husband, Doug, who typed and edited the manuscript I wrote by hand; and who tirelessly supported me through this process.

To Dr. Robert Curry, whose editorial insights helped make this manuscript more cohesive, and whose support and leadership over the years have inspired me to keep learning.

AUTHOR'S NOTE

This booklet is based on the following principles:

1. I don't claim to know everything.
2. You and I are always learning.
3. This book is a compilation of numerous medical and nutritional studies which I have read and want to share with you.
4. You and I are fellow travelers on the road to health and wellness.

Mary Frost has a B.A. in Journalism from the University of Texas and a Masters of Arts and Liberal Arts from St. Johns College (The Great Books Program). She has been actively involved in health and nutrition for more than 15 years and brings her experience and studies to the fore as a nutritional journalist.

This booklet is intended for educational purposes only, and should not be used as a guide for diagnosis or treatment of any kind.

Table of Contents

Introduction—Why Whole Food Supplements?

Most of us have gotten used to reading literature proclaiming the benefits of vitamins, deciding what is wrong with us, and heading to the health food store to buy what we have decided we need. Often, we end up buying all kinds of supplements and, **we are still not any healthier.**

I was a health food store junkie myself before I found a health professional who tested me for what I needed. I was getting frequent sinus infections (7 in 2 years) that always resulted in laryngitis. I was taking Vitamin A (25,000iu), Vitamin E (400iu), ascorbic acid with rosehips (3,000mg), Kyolic garlic, echinacea, golden seal, and homeopathics, and **they were not helping.** Truthfully, I was afraid that my immune system was weakening, and I had visions of dying of pneumonia.

Fortunately, I found a health professional who determined what my health problem was, and got me started on some supplements from Standard Process, a company that has manufactured whole food supplements since 1929. I do not get sick anymore. If I start to get the sniffles, I take some Standard Process supplements and I am quickly over them. Before, I would take the protocol mentioned above and I would still get sick. I could not prevent it.

What I have come to realize, over the years that I have been with Standard Process, is that **we cannot understand what this company offers** in the way of nutritional supplements **unless we understand what has happened, step by step, to our food supply,** and we cannot understand what Standard Process is **unless we understand what most vitamins today really are.**

For years Americans have gotten used to the "new and improved" idea. We don't even know what the truth is. We don't know how to step back and evaluate whether the information being advertised is a fad or not. We are told not to eat butter, eat margarine instead. Then 20 years later we are told that margarine is a trans-fatty acid and dangerous for us. We are told not to eat eggs or beef because they can cause cholesterol problems, then years later we are told that they are OK.

So, we are presented with "new medical facts" that are advertised in such a way as to persuade us to change our eating habits and go in a different direction. What we are getting is what Ralph Nader calls "pseudo-science". And what we are getting are genetically engineered foods, faulty infomercial health tips, incorrect information about what we are already eating, and tricky nutritional labels that we have no way of deciphering.

We need to stop listening to what Dr. Bernard Jensen and Mark Anderson call "those television advertising managers practicing medicine without a brain". This booklet is an attempt to pull back the camouflage and look at the inner workings of this gigantic mess. This will show why we must tune out the antacid and the low-fat diet food commercials, and why we must watch out for synthetic vitamins by themselves or hidden in an herbal formula or an aromatherapy oil. This booklet is a guide to know how to evaluate all this and stay healthy.

Standard Process has always been available **only through health professionals.** Most people come to Standard Process in desperation. Accustomed to reading labels, very little on the bottles makes sense to them. But after a while of taking the specific supplements they were tested to need, most people are amazed at the difference and want to know more.

In the years that I have been with Standard Process, I have seen amazing results with all kinds of problems that people present to me. Standard Process products really help to build the immune system and make people stronger and healthier.

But taking Standard Process products wasn't all that I needed, because eating a low-fat diet had me tired and fatigued most of the time and I couldn't figure it out. Someone introduced me to Jay Robb's <u>Fat Burning Diet</u> and, **within a short time,** I felt my life force coming back. It was then that I realized the importance of blood sugar and optimum health. I read everything I could get my hands on about this, which led me to the book, <u>Protein Power</u>, I quote extensively here. This book leaves no stone unturned in exposing the deadly issue of excessive insulin in the body.

I hope you enjoy reading this information — and that it opens your eyes to what the **real issues of health in America today really are.**

I go into these issues in a lot more depth in my next book, <u>The Biggest Cover-up of the 20th Century</u>.

> Thus we should beware of clinging to
> vulgar opinions, and judge things by
> reason's way, not by popular say.
>
> *Montaigne* (1533–1592)

Health Crisis

Today, Americans are in a health crisis. Statistics abound:

*3 out of every 4 Americans will get heart disease — 2 out of every 4 will die from it.

*According to the American Diabetes Association, the number of diabetics has increased from 6 to 16 million in the last 15 years, and another 21 million have *"impaired glucose tolerance."*

*Some form of depression, anxiety, or fatigue affects over 50% of the population.

*200,000 Americans die yearly from high blood pressure and stroke.

*Roughly 25% of all adult Americans are *"significantly overweight."*

From these statistics, if you filled a Boeing 747 Jumbo Jet to capacity (300 people) and computed into airline crashes the number of deaths resulting from heart disease, hypertension, and diabetes, you would have 3,650 Jumbo Jet crashes a year! That would be 10 Jumbo Jets falling out of the sky every day!

How many of us would fly again with such risks involved? It is pretty sick thinking, but it creates what scholars have named the "outrage" factor: (how people react differently to death or disability from a specific cause).

And outraged is what we as a nation should be! But we are more concerned when a plane crashes because of the publicity than we are of the number of people dying from heart disease every year. Yet, there is a lot of human misery reflected in these frightening statistics, plus the billions of dollars involved in the health care needs these people require. Orthodox Medical Care spending is now estimated at $200 billion.

What to Do?

In the attempt to protect themselves and their families from these frightening occurences, Americans are changing their diets and are taking herbs and supplements. The money spent on the Alternative Health Industry is estimated at over $1 billion this past year. Over-the-counter vitamin sales are at $9 billion. **This means that most people buy their vitamins from a store clerk!!!**

And yet, people are getting sicker. They pump vitamins and eat "right", but that does not seem to be the answer. They are still fatigued, still overweight, still fighting the cholesterol battle, etc..., etc...

Nearly every week, my clients and I get at least 2 or 3 mailers touting some "New Medical Cure" or "Amazing Discoveries". It was in response to this deluge of material that my clients have urged me to write this booklet— **To enable people to wade** through all this information and make an informed decision.

What is Wrong with This Picture?

When people are trying so hard to do the right thing, why aren't the results long-term? Why do they feel so great when they start taking vitamins and later feel fatigued again? *Why are 95% of the people who lose weight unable to keep it off?* Why are the statistics on heart disease, hypertension, and diabetes getting worse?

My studies have left me to conclude that the 3 major culprits are:

1) **The harm that is done to our food before it even gets to us.** The depletion and demineralization of America's topsoil, the contamination of produce by excessive use of pesticides and fungicides, the chemicalization of food through over-processing, enriching, preserving, and the contamination of water through fluoridation

2) **Synthetic vitamins taken as supplements**

3) **Low-Fat, Low-Protein, High-Carbohydrate Diets**

Where Do We Start?

Foods are not what they seem anymore. Consider these facts:

*In order to get the iron that was available in one cup of spinach in 1945, you would have to consume **65** cups today.

*An orange that contained 50mg of natural vitamin C complex in 1950 now contains **5mg.**

In most instances, that lovely green salad on your table is practically dead nutritionally!

We are producing less nutritious food at the highest cost in history while United States farmers are going bankrupt. (1)

How can this be? America's topsoil has been depleted through:

1) Deforestation

2) Incorrect Farming Methods

3) Overuse of Fungicides and Pesticides

Deforestation

Deforestation, while not in itself responsible for our nutritionally-dead foods, marks the first major assault in the ***dismantling of our natural ecosystem.*** The cutting down of massive amounts of trees "laid bare" a disrespect for Mother Nature **and a lack of interest in Her inner workings** that paved the way for our lack of health today.

When settlers began arriving in America in the 16th century, they found a land in pristine condition.

After thousands of years of use by Native Americans, the water was still pure. The land was so fertile, that if you dropped a seed on it, it would grow. Trees and forests were everywhere. In fact, in the Iroquoi Nation folklore, they would speak of how a squirrel could hop from tree to tree from the Atlantic Ocean to the Mississippi River! When they gave directions, "grandfather trees" were used as landmarks.

Today, we are lucky to have any good topsoil, or any forests at all.

> In Iowa, topsoils that were once a foot deep, today are less than six inches deep. Although it doesn't sound like much, six inches can be devastating. The United States Department of Agriculture estimates that a six-inch loss of topsoil, such as the current one in the southern Piedmont, is capable of reducing crop yields by 40% per year. (2)

The European settlers of this country found 18 to 25 inches of rich topsoil in the 1700's. Now, most farmlands are like those in Iowa. In fact, the dust storms that occured in the 1930's in Kansas *that left topsoil on desktops in Washington D.C.* are about to return-- statistics say that in 1977, 5 million acres were severely eroded by wind, and by 1988 estimates were at 25 million acres. (Areas **double** the size of Maryland and Massachusetts **combined.**)

> Kansas Congressman Dan Glickman stated in March of 1989, 'It's no secret the central

part of America is blowing away right now'. (3)

The natural trees, grasses, and vegetation that once anchored the soil are gone. To date, over **260 million acres of trees in America** have been cut to make way for raising livestock! *Trees shade the soil, hold the soil in place, and act as pumps to draw water up near the surface of the ground, thus keeping water tables high.* Without trees, the soil gets baked dry by the sun, and eventually gets blown away by the wind or wasted away by rains.

West Texas was once covered with tall grasses; now it is a flat, barren area where high winds carrying loose soil can turn the sky black. Over-grazing cattle pulled these grasses out of the soil, leaving nothing to hold it in place.

When you see all of the starving people in East Africa, what you are seeing is famine caused by a land laid bare through deforestation. In Ethiopia, for example, 90% of the land was covered by forests in 1890 — now barely **5%** remains. Environmentalists, realizing this, have tried to stop the current destruction of the Brazilian rainforests, but the massive cutting down of trees continues. America's National Parks, our last forest reserves, are being threatened today by adjacent mining activities, clear-cutting, oil and gas exploration, and many other related activities.

Incorrect Farming Methods

The massive use of chemical fertilizers, which are manufactured and shipped around the world by the millions of tons per year, has come to be an accepted method of **forcing plants to grow.** This method was conceived in a paper published by the renowned German chemist, Baron Justus von Liebig, in 1855. In this document, von Liebig determined that the only minerals plants needed were nitrogen, phosphorus, and potassium.

The German chemical industry flourished on this premise, and agressively marketed it to farmers. The imbalance in trace minerals, fungus, and microbial life that this "artificial manure" created was later regretted by von Liebig. At the end of his life, he wrote, **"Nature herself points...out to man the proper course of proceeding for keeping up the productiveness of the land."** (4)

Some 20 years later after von Liebig's death, the famed German naturalist Julius Hensel ridiculed this nitrogen-phosphorus-potassium theory and encouraged farmers to spread a finely crushed, **minerally rich rock dust** on their land. "Those who did were amazed at the quality, strength, and drought resistancy of their crops." (5)

The thriving chemical industrialists were so vicious and vigorous in their attempt to discredit Hensel that **his book could not be found anywhere for many years.**

The high-handed techniques used by the chemical industrialists illustrate how an idea that went against economic interests of the time could be squelched with such *ferocity that the consumers (in this case, the farmers) were led to conclude that it was false.*

In 1940, Sir Albert Howard published his landmark book, <u>An Agricultural Testament</u>. In it he promoted Hensel's rock dust theories and gave a sobering warning about the use of chemical fertilizers:

> The principle followed, based on the von Liebig tradition, is that any deficiencies in the soil can be made up by the addition of suitable chemicals (man-made). This is based on a complete misconception of plant nutrition. It is superficial and fundamentally unsound. It takes no account of the life of the soil, including mycorrhizal association- the living fungus bridge which connects the soil and sap. **Artificial manures lead inevitably to artificial nutrition, artificial food, artificial animals, and finally, to artificial men and women.** (6)

These chemical fertilizers kill most of the microorganisms and worms in the topsoil, then they trickle down through the ground to contaminate underground water supplies. In 1989, the Nutrient Testing Laboratory ran mineral analysis tests on commercial produce from regions around the United States: **Sodium levels were high** in all produce tested, while many other trace elements were not even present. The reason for this is because chemical fertilizers are highly concentrated inorganic salts.

Fungicides and Pesticides Are Not Working

Farming has become a high tech industry, combining technology and economics to exploit the land they farm for profit. "The result: *modern agriculture reduces the role of soil to a substance of convenient texture that holds plants in the vertical position while chemicals are forced up their shaft. Plants stand in the field and receive a chemical enema.*" (7)

> The modern farmer looks down from the air-conditioned cab of his $100,000 John Deere tractor and says 'What's this?' He sees a little fungus growing on the plant and he says, 'We aren't going to put up with this. We know how to deal with the likes of you!'
>
> He gets into his pickup truck, heads down to the agriculture chemical supply station, and returns loaded with barrels of chemosterilants, with skull and crossbones on their labels. Now he is ready to treat the plant. In the back of his pickup truck are barrels with labels that say things like: *'Use extreme caution— do not inhale—use in well-ventilated areas—do not allow any contact with skin and hair—do not dispose near water— keep away from livestock and feed—may cause blindness or death if taken internally—read all instructions carefully—federal law requires application*

in accordance with label data', and he thinks, 'This looks good. Let's apply this to our growing food.' (8)

Land that once was fertile in the Mississippi Delta is so devoid of worms (a sign of healthy soil) and other microbiotic life that the remains of harvested crops cannot be turned under any more. This is due to so many years of soil sterilization that ***the soil is now incapable of even rotting and composting.***

Pesticide production from 1947 to 1960 increased from 259,000 pounds per year to almost 6.4 million pounds! **Yet, "Crop loss due to insect damage has *doubled* since World War II,** from 7% to 14%." (9)

Insecticides are so deadly, that one form, *Zyklan B,* was what the Nazis used to gas millions of their victims in the concentration camps from 1939 to1945. Another, *Methyl Isocyanate,* caused the death of over 3,500 people in Bhopal, India, and maimed 200,000 more.

Pesticide residues can be found in plants grown in soil previously sprayed years before. In fact, organic farmers in California deal with "Certified Organic" labeling as follows: No chemical fertilizers or pesticides/fungicides can be used on the land for 3 years, and the land is built-up organically. At the end of those 3 years, the produce is tested for pesticide residue. If there is any, the farmer must wait another year and have his produce tested again before he can label it "Certified Organic".

You would think that the failure of pesticides to eliminate crop damage would cause these chemical companies to look at possibly contributing to a natural solution. Not so. <u>Mother Jones</u>, in its Jan/Feb 1997 issue, did an article on <u>The Future of Food</u>. From potato and corn seeds that are **genetically altered** to have a built-in pesticide to soybean seeds that are **genetically manipulated** to survive direct applications of Roundup (so that the manufacturer can sell more), these companies are on **a destructive track.** The article did ask an important question: *"Is anyone protecting the consumers?"*

Soil is a Living Substance

Soil is the basis of all life. The plants that grow in soil are the food for the animals on the lowest end of the food chain. These animals are the the food supply for the animals at the highest end of the chain.

William Albrecht, PhD, of the University of Missouri, found that he could cure undulent fever in livestock and humans by adding trace minerals to the soil in which their food was grown (Henry Ford's only son, Edsel, died from undulent fever.). Albrecht proved that mineral deficiencies and agri-chemical toxicity caused plant vulnerability to fungus, drought, insects, and disease in general.

Good soil is composed of 45% minerals and millions of microorganisms. Dr. Albrecht and Dr. Royal Lee, founder of Standard Process, were adamant about this:

> When we see a symptom in the plant, it will always correlate to a poison or deficiency in the soil; when we see a disease in the human, it will relate to a poison or deficiency in the food. (10)

Mineral-deficient soil is targeted as one of the original sources of disease in the world today.

Simply stated, food crops grown on
depleted soil produce malnourished
bodies, and disease preys on malnourished
bodies. (11)

How Does A Plant Protect Itself?

What these high tech farmers are lacking is true understanding of the plant's immune system. At the root system, little offshoots called rootlets have hair-like fungi growing on them called *mycorrhiza.*

Mineral-rich soil has millions of microorganisms living in it, and their primary function is to decompose anything that falls on the land, and to break down mineral deposits into plant food. The plant doesn't get devoured by these organisms (bacteria) because the *mycorrhiza* secretes antibiotics to protect the plant (Keep in mind that penicillin comes from a fungus).

Nature gave fungi and bacteria an
interesting relationship. They are natural
antagonists. They keep each other in check
through their competition …the plant, thus
protected, is free to absorb the minerals
that soil microbial life has released without
fear of infection from soil-borne bacteria. (12)

If you see a fungus growing on a plant, it is a self-produced fungus because there was something inferior about the quality of the plant. Nature grows fungus on the inferior plant, then it dies, decomposes, and begins again—until it gets it right.

The Importance of Trace Minerals

"Human bodies require nutrition found in the form of plants, meat, milk, and eggs." (13) Since animals get their food directly or indirectly from plants, and plants get their food from the soil, there is a direct link to human health from the soil.

Much is now said in the news media of the importance of different trace minerals such as selenium, boron, chromium etc.... But just the absence of one mineral can cause great health problems.

*Without the trace mineral cobalt, the human body cannot manufacture B12.

*Without potassium, the heart muscle can be harmed, and the result can be a racing of the heartbeat or tachycardia.

*Without zinc, selenium, sulfur, and iron, the liver would be sluggish and/or weak in its ability to repair damaged tissue, fight infection, and detoxify the blood and the bowel.

Remember, plants do not manufacture trace minerals, they **absorb them.** The health of the soil's microbial life depends upon the trace minerals in the soil, and so do *enzymes,* the most important ingredient in plant, animal, and human biochemistry. All metabolic processes at every level depend on enzymes.

Often, enzymes vital to our immune systems need the rarest trace minerals in order to function.

There are **92 known trace elements.** As research continues, it is reasonable to assume that the role of every mineral will be discovered, with the notable exception of **lead, aluminium, cadmium, and mercury, which are toxic.**

Dr. Wallach, in his tape <u>Dead Doctors Don't Lie</u>, expounds the importance of trace minerals. I totally agree with him. The source he recommends comes from fossilized prehistoric plant life, but **contains aluminium and cadmium,** as stated on the label. Standard Process's All-Organic Trace Minerals ***does not*** contain aluminium or cadmium. Dr. Royal Lee, in his foresight, chose the location for Standard Process's farms in a rich, fertile area known as the Kettle Morraine, which was formed by retreating glaciers in the last Ice Age. *All* Standard Process products are harvested with all trace minerals intact.

Let's Get Real

As we drive in our air-conditioned cars to our air-conditioned office and sit down in front of our computers — only to go home at night and sit in front of the TV, we are prey to an assault of information unparalleled in history. Yet, so much of what we hear does not take total, ***factual information*** into account. (See the Atlas of Planetary Management on the next 2 pages)

The advocates of whole foods and organic farming are so out-talked by advocates of big business that we can hardly hear the truth through all of their

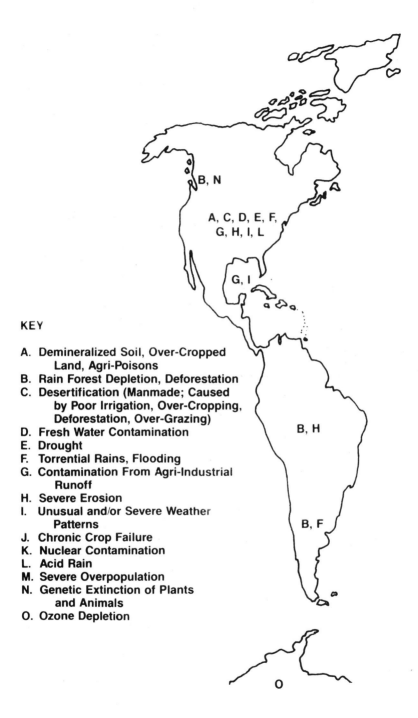

B, N

A, C, D, E, F,
G, H, I, L

G, I

KEY

A. Demineralized Soil, Over-Cropped
   Land, Agri-Poisons
B. Rain Forest Depletion, Deforestation
C. Desertification (Manmade; Caused
   by Poor Irrigation, Over-Cropping,
   Deforestation, Over-Grazing)
D. Fresh Water Contamination
E. Drought
F. Torrential Rains, Flooding
G. Contamination From Agri-Industrial
   Runoff
H. Severe Erosion
I. Unusual and/or Severe Weather
   Patterns
J. Chronic Crop Failure
K. Nuclear Contamination
L. Acid Rain
M. Severe Overpopulation
N. Genetic Extinction of Plants
   and Animals
O. Ozone Depletion

B, H

B, F

O

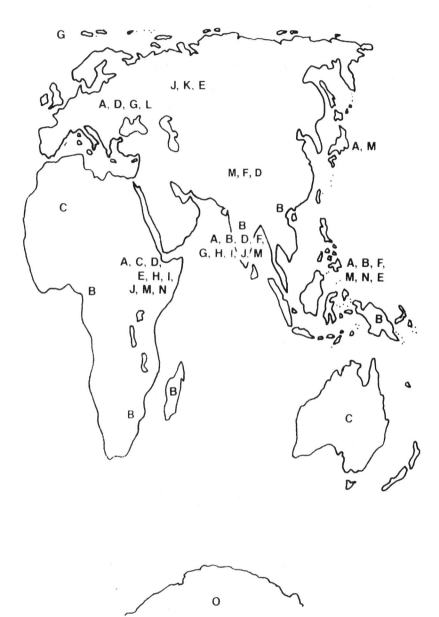

O

G

J, K, E

A, D, G, L

A, M

M, F, D

C

B

B

A, B, D, F,
G, H, I, J, M

A, B, F,
M, N, E

A, C, D,
E, H, I,
J, M, N

B

B

B

B

C

O

blaring. But our bodies know what is happening. The innate intelligence in our bodies is telling us through heart disease, cancer, AIDS, diabetes, and obesity that something is amiss. And our souls are telling us that profits aren't everything.

> Although the popular ecology movement grabs an occasional headline, what our political leaders, scientists, and doctors are unwilling to come to grips with is that we are on the threshold of vast human annihilation. (14)

Consider what historian V.G. Simkovich had to say about the ruins of ancient civilizations:

> Look at the unpeopled valleys, at the dead and buried cities, and you can decipher there the promise and the prophecy of us.... Depleted of humus by constant cropping, land could no longer reward labor and support life, so the people abandoned it. Deserted, it became a desert; the light soil was washed by the rain and blown around by the shifting winds. (15)

There is a possibilty to reverse this trend. John D. Hamaker, in his monumental work, <u>The Survival of Civilization</u>, does give us some guidelines.

> Hamaker believes that an all-out global effort to remineralize the Earth's soils (with rock dust) and the planting of billions of trees, coupled with the

elimination of fossil fuel burning, and the developement of alternative sources of power (for example, hydrogen, solar, and wind) can restore the carbon balance between the land and atmosphere. (16)

The Chemicalization of Foods

So, we have chopped down millions of acres of trees, over-grazed millions of acres of natural vegetation, poured chemical fertilizers on the soil, and sprayed the plants with fungicides and pesticides. **Now, *the stage is set to really attack our food supply in earnest!*** Since whole, natural foods tend to decay or go rancid quickly, methods for producing a long shelf life went into high gear.

When we walk through a grocery store and read labels, it can be a journey through a *chemical laboratory.* All the contents have preservatives, additives, and synthetic vitamins that we have just come to take for granted. The shocking truth of how all these substances came to be in our foods is not fully understood, but should be.

As Dr. Bernard Jensen and Mark Anderson pointed out in their book, Empty Harvest, within a generation following World War I, the **foods of commerce** took over.

The food supply became bleached, refined, chemically preserved, pasteurized, sterilized, homogenized, hydrogenated, artificially colored, defibered, highly sugared, highly salted, synthetically fortified (enriched), canned, and generally exposed to hundreds of new man-made chemicals. (17)

How did this happen? Where was the **Food and Drug Administration?** The Pure Food and Drug Law was subverted and manipulated by commercial interests starting in 1912. At that time, these commercial interests forced Dr. Harvey W. Wiley from his office as founder and head of the Bureau of Chemistry, now known as the FDA. As you can see in the cartoon on the next page, Dr. Wiley's departure was seen as an open frolic of synthetic food enhancers.

When he had filed suit against Coca-Cola to keep this artificial product off the market and prohibit its interstate transport, Dr. Wiley said:

> No food product in our country would have any trace of benzoic acid, sulfurous acid or sulfites or any alum or saccharin, save for medical purposes. No soft drink would contain caffeine or theobromine. No bleached flour would enter interstate commerce. Our foods and drugs would be wholly without any form of adulteration and misbranding. The health of our people would be vastly improved and the life greatly extended. The manufacturers of our food supply, and especially the millers, would devote their energies to improving the public health and promoting happiness in every home by the production of whole ground, unbolted cereal flours and meals. (18)

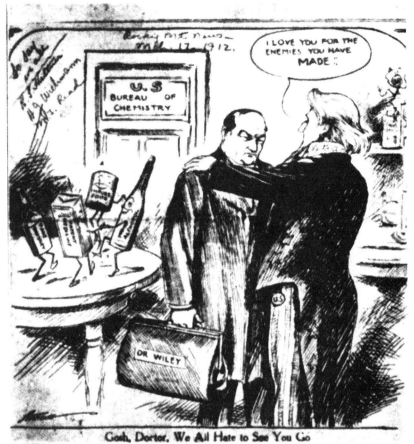

Source: *Rocky Mountain News*, c. March 1912

Cartoons Depict Reaction to Dr. Wiley's Departure From
Bureau of Chemistry

Above, as Dr. Wiley prepares to leave, on the table behind him, impure foods,
patent medicines, and ersatz substances hold hands and dance for joy. Above
right, Uncle Sam bids farewell, and laments the end of Dr. Wiley's career at
the Bureau of Chemistry.

Photo and caption by permission of Mark Anderson

A Dark Period for the FDA Begins

Dr. Wiley's departure led the way for a replacement in the form of Dr. Elmer M. Nelson, a commercially-backed man placed in the front line of all decision-making.

The following is a quote from Dr. Nelson's testimony given in federal court to block health food manufacturers from comparing the quality of their products to their synthetic, processed counterparts.

> *It is wholly unscientific to state that a well-fed body is more able to resist disease than a less well-fed body.* My overall opinion is that there hasn't been enough experimentation to prove dietary deficiencies make one more susceptible to disease. (19)

Unbelievable? Incredible? How many people today know that dietary deficiencies can lead to degenerative diseases, infectious diseases, and functional diseases? The American public has been the official testing "lab" for this kind of fallacious thinking, and *it was this kind of reasoning that Dr. Nelson and his team of "experts" expounded for over 10 years in court to get the OK on the synthetics that we have in foods today.*

It is important to note that landmark works in nutrition by Dr. Weston Price, Dr. Francis Pottenger, Dr. Roger Williams, Dr. Agnes Fay Morgan, and Dr. Royal Lee were totally **ignored and treated with disdain.**

The truth was helpless in the face of an FDA that had unlimited taxpayer dollars at its disposal to promote the commercial interests of the time.

The Persecution of Dr. Lee

> ...we must not assume that science and truth march straight ahead and that the present is the beneficiary of the accumulated knowledge of the past. Because, in many instances—and health and nutrition is one—**the past is full of deception and factual manipulation** resulting in the inheritance of a tarnished view of scientific progess.
>
> <u>Empty Harvest</u>

Dr. Royal Lee, founder of Standard Process, was a pioneer in the field of nutrition (some consider him the world's greatest nutritionist). **His processing techniques are even today so far beyond what anyone else is doing in the supplement industry as to seem an undreamed of possibility.**

Dr. Lee's genius as an electronic inventor led to more than 100 electronic patents (such as the governor for electric motors and the Phono-Cardiograph). He invented advanced weapons control systems during WWII, and he assisted NASA with his motor control design for their Lunar Guidance Systems. However, Dr. Lee's overwhelming passion was nutrition. He incorporated Dr. Albrecht's experiments and discoveries with soil into his own research; and, for almost 50 years, Dr. Lee "amassed an encyclopedic body of knowledge in plant, animal, and human health and its links to soil, food processing, diet, and nutrition…. To coordinate and communicate nutritional breakthroughs from both his own laboratory and laboratories throughout the world, he established The Lee Foundation for Nutritional Research, which in its day was the world's largest clearing house for nutritional information for doctors, homemakers, and agriculturalists." (20)

In 1937, at the same time Dr. Lee was in court fighting the FDA to be able to advertise Zypan (the hydrochloric acid tablet he designed to help with digestion), Camel cigarettes was able to advertise in <u>Life</u> magazine that smoking cigarettes would promote digestion!!! This Camel ad can be seen in <u>Empty Harvest</u> and it shows a Thanksgiving meal divided into five courses, with short blurbs on how smoking in between each course will "help your digestion to run smoothly". (21) A food editor, Miss Dorothy Malone, is pictured in one corner of the ad, saying, "It's smart to have Camels on the table. My own personal experience is that smoking Camels with my meals and afterwards builds up a sense of digestive well-being." (22) The cigarette ad went on to say, "Enjoy Camels all you wish— all through the day." (23)

How many people were powerfully persuaded to smoke cigarettes because of advertising? Many people feel that if it is advertised, it is gospel. Advertising creates fads and trends. Today, cigarette companies would never be allowed to make such claims. Hundreds of thousands of people with lung cancer and emphysema followed this type of advertising advice.

What about another ad, from 1955, reported in Empty Harvest, that claims that "Science shows how sugar can help keep your appetite—and weight—under control." (24) This ad actually promoted elevating blood sugar to cut down the sensation of hunger. Millions of people have become diabetics following such fallacious advice.

Yet, during the years that these and many other misleading ads were allowed to be printed by the FDA, Dr. Lee was constantly in Federal Court, trying to get *the right to advertise his nutritional products!* If this sounds upside down, it is!

> …Dr. Lee and other pioneers exposed the chronic malnutrition rampant in our nation, how indigestion was caused by the worn-out digestive tracts of the civilized diet, how dental caries, diabetes, and other diseases were caused by sugar, and they were persecuted with the full power and unlimited taxpayer resources of the FDA. **Dr. Lee was branded a racketeer because he promoted whole, natural, unadulterated foods** with their vitamins and minerals intact. When he designed digestive aids with enzymes and calcium products to replace the loss of the minerals through processing and sugarized diets, he was branded a faddist and extremist who was duping the public. (25)

Dr. Lee was trying to give the public a way of getting the vitamins and other nutrients that were removed from flour and rice by commercial milling. He knew that these factors were the reason for the epidemic of coronary heart attacks that was sweeping the country in the early 1920's. And every time he tried to advertise anything that related to what was going on, he ended up in court.

As Dr. Lee's and other's voices got muffled out, the marketplace became filled with grains and cereals that had artificial vitamins added back into them, all for huge profits.

> The newsletter of The Center for Science in the Public Interest, *Nutritional Action* (Vol. 16, No. 1), reports that the only difference between General Mills' Wheaties and Total cereals is that 1.5 cents' worth of synthetic vitamins are sprayed on Total. Total is then sold for 65 cents more than Wheaties. This practice alone has generated **$425 million** in additional profits since 1972 for General Mills. (26)

Sadly, these huge profits mean that millions of people have ingested untold pounds of chemicalized and enriched food. Sadly also, the world that Dr. Wiley, Dr. Lee, and others envisioned was not allowed to be.

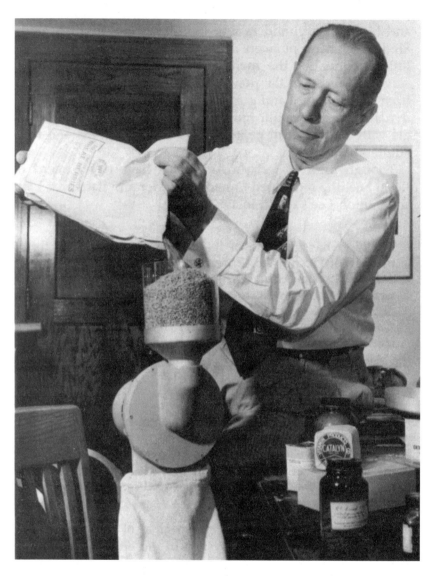

Dr. Royal Lee (1895–1967)

Perhaps the world's greatest nutritionist, Dr. Lee was also a prolific electronic inventor. Here he is working on his famous Lee Flour Mill. He designed it so the average household could have wholesome, fresh, low-heat, stone-ground flour with the vitamin-rich germ and fiber-full bran intact. His Lee Foundation for Nutritional Research was a lighthouse as food adulteration and commercialism swept the twentieth century.

Photo and caption by permission of Mark Anderson

A Word or Two About Oils

One hundred years ago, heart attacks were practically unheard of in the U.S. The first recorded case of atherosclerosis was in 1910; the first reported heart attack was in 1912. **Alzheimer's disease did not exist. One person in 100,000 had diabetes, and in Europe, cancer caused 3.4% of all deaths. Now about two-thirds of Americans develop atherosclerosis; 50% die of cardiovascular disease. Alzheimer's is the fourth leading cause of death. One in 20 has some form of diabetes. One in four (28%) develops cancer—500,000 of them die.** Other degenerative conditions which have exploded in numbers since the turn of the century include multiple sclerosis, kidney degeneration, liver degeneration, and others. **One hundred years ago, people ate fresh, whole foods including plenty of meat, butter, and lard. But they did not ordinarily eat any refined, processed, or chemicalized foods, did not eat any refined and altered oils or fats. All these are now commonly consumed.** (27)

Many of the steps used to process vegetable oils can affect the nutritional content and balance of these products. Expeller-pressed oils and hydraulic-pressed oils are first subjected to temperatures of 200 degrees F and up. The oils are then de-gummed, which removes chlorophyll, vitamin E, lecithin, and many minerals and trace elements. Then an alkaline wash seperates out even even more nutrients. Next, the oil is bleached and then deodorized by steam distillation at temperatures over 450 degrees F.

> The resulting oil is colorless, tasteless, odorless, altered, and, of course, devoid of nutrients. Any vitamin complexes in the original food are gone; any possible remnants of nutrients are only fractions. (28)

Since the FDA has established **no legal meaning** for the term "cold pressed", a manufacturer can use the term on labels, even if the oil has been heated, degummed, bleached, refined, or otherwise chemically altered.

Poisons Found in Refined Oils

The raw materials for oils now come from large, chemically-farmed fields. Very often, these over-refined oils contain pesticide residue, which interferes with nerve function and oxidation processes in the human body. **These pesticide residues are only some of the toxic substances that are found in altered oils.**

Trans-fatty acids, **another toxic substance,** make up, on the average, almost 10% of the total fats in the American Diet. Trans-fatty acids are made by forcing hydrogen into raw, polyunsaturated oil molecules under high temperature and pressure. The oil is chemically altered so that the oil is more solid and has a longer shelf life.

People are encouraged to eat low fat. They avoid animal products and consume large quantities of margarine, cookies, cake, and white bread, which greatly increases their intake of trans-fatty acids.

> Nutritional researcher, John Finnegan, states: 'There is more and more evidence showing that the main cause of heart disease and one of the main causes of cancer is the harmful effects from poisonous trans-fats and other compounds in refined oils.' (29)

If you are confused as to how to identify trans-fatty acids, here are the key markers:

1) **The words "partially hydrogenated" in the list of ingredients on a product.**

2) **Oil that is packaged in a clear bottle. Sunlight can penetrate and cause the oils to go rancid.** Unfortunately, you will even find these in most health food stores, where almost all "are usually manufactured by the same refineries as supermarket oils." (30) **Buy oil in cans or dark brown glass bottles.**

3) **Oils that are odorless and tasteless.** Fresh, natural oils have their own delicate flavor and aroma.

We need the unsaturated fatty acids from good oils for many reasons: **healthy skin and hair, maintenance of normal growth, hormone production, proper digestion, wound healing, calcium metabolism, etc....** Obviously, we have to be careful to choose good oils to get the job done.

<u>Water — The Crucial Commodity</u>

Both the endocrine system and the immune system are the most vitamin and mineral dependent of all the systems in our bodies. One of the worst poisons our glands can encounter, *sodium fluoride,* is now added to most municipal drinking water. Calcium fluoride, a natural form of fluoride found in trace amounts in well water, was *not,* unfortunately, chosen by the municipalities. **Sodium fluoride is a highly toxic by-product of aluminium production and can destroy the enzymes that make vitamins work in your body!**

Dr. Lee was one of the first informed opponents to fluoridation. He called it "an attempt to treat a deficiency disease (dental caries), a case of starvation, with a poisonous drug." (31) In fact, Dr. Lee developed the first patent for making protein-bound iodine so that one can ingest it orally and not burn the stomach.

Protein-bound iodine is a very important radiation protective factor. Your body makes thyroxin out of it, and if you are deficient in it, your body may try to make thyroxin out of the next closest material, sodium fluoride, another halogen molecule. This then weakens the thyroid.

Non-fluoridated cities across the U.S. have had the same amount of dental caries as those cities that are fluoridated (<u>Chemical and Engineering News</u>, August 1, 1988)!! Americans have been **forced to medicate their public water,** yet studies have shown over and over again, *it not only does not prevent caries, but it is toxic!*

The thyroid, the endocrine gland of metabolism, helps the body adapt between heat and cold. Most people have such unresponsive thyroids that their bodies do not respond appropriately to the temperature changes that winter brings. A weak thyroid **results in unprocessed metabolic waste accumulating in the system.** When this waste-loaded lymph backs up into the sytem or lymph nodes, the bowel becomes sluggish.

Many naturalist doctors agree that as the metabolic waste continues to build up, the person gets the flu or a cold. The flu is a violent detoxification process that helps the body get rid of its wastes. A cold is a case of the bacteria living on the unprocessed metabolic waste.

So, whatever you do, supporting your thyroid nutritionally has become necessary for optimum health.

Synthetic Vitamins Taken as Supplements

With such an unethical beginning, the FDA has left the public with a commercial food industry staggering in its size and revenues, and a health care crisis that is *out of control.*

Now we have our food supply thoroughly corrupted and polluted. In an effort to help themselves, people take "natural" and "organic" supplements.

But the truth is, when you purchase these products, you are merely getting more of what is being dumped into our food supply!!!

Thiamine HCL and Thiamine Mononitrate as B1 come from **coal tar;** d-alpha tocopherols as Vitamin E are fractions extracted from **processed and refined food oils** (mainly cottonseed and soybean oil); dl-alpha tocopherols are **manufactured in a laboratory;** and ascorbic acid as Vitamin C is made from **refined corn sugar,** just to name a few.

How did this happen? What *exactly* do the terms "natural" and "organic" mean according to the FDA?

*Natural— anything that ultimately comes from nature, including chemicals, since they ultimately come from nature

*Organic— anything that contains a carbon molecule (DDT has a carbon base)

By leaving these terms basically undefined, our imagination is left to "fill in the blanks". Is this what we had in mind when we purchased a "natural" vitamin, or an "organic" supplement? Imagine a farm where no pesticides are used and the land is fertilized with composting? Well, *that is not the way it is.*

Why Natural Food Complexes Faded From View

In the beginning of vitamin research, almost all of the scientific experiments used natural, food-sourced nutrients, and a lot was learned. Nutrients are difficult for the FDA and other agencies to control. But isolating vitamins and standardizing them as drugs gives them a **means of controlling them.**

> For the pharmaceutical companies, vitamin fractions such as 'Vitamins' A, C, beta-carotene, and E; trace minerals as zinc and selenium (usually sold in inorganic and imbalanced forms), coenzyme Q, and many other specific nutrients can be cheaply manufactured and sold at huge profits. (32)

Judith DeCava, in her book <u>The Real Truth About Vitamins and Antioxidants</u>, talks about the "standard medical view", which is an "attempt to blend medicine with nutrition, using chemically-isolated nutrients as drugs." DeCava makes some important points:

1) "**Medical schools in this country are now standardized** (if not homogenized) and no matter what medical school one attends, one gets essentially the same instruction..." (83)

2) "**Doctors believe that their education gives them a strange sort of infallability to lend their expertise in areas of medicine for which they have received *no training,*** as in nutrition, leading them to discount ideas and even valid research." (84) This is supported by the fact that in 1991, only 22 out of the 127 accredited U.S. Medical Schools *required a single course in nutrition.*

3) **"News of nutrients from 1962 onward—** whether in medical journals, newspapers, TV, radio- are nearly or entirely all based on studies using the fractionated, crystalline-pure, synthetic chemicals. The obvious consequence follows: **The nutrition industry has turned into a money-grabbing, hustling, lying, cheating scam,** as described by a sales rep of a very reputable supplement company." (33)

Cellular malnutrition as a cause of diseases has been drifted away from in orthodox medicine, and synthetic vitamins, which have druglike effects, have been embraced. Often, these synthetics actually contaminate the internal environment of the body. But these synthetics, unlike whole food concentrates, can be easily mass-produced by large pharmaceutical companies, who can store and distribute them. As a result, these isolated synthetics are used in nearly all nutritional supplements, whether found in a drug store, health food store, or nutritionist's office.

Just What are Natural Complexes?

Vitamins are "groups of chemically related compounds". There is a part that is identified as the organic nutrient of the vitamin, i.e., ascorbic acid as Vitamin C. **But then there are enzymes, coenzymes, antioxidants, trace elements, activators, and other unknown factors that enable the vitamin to go into biochemical operation** (See diagrams on the next 2 pages).

−34−

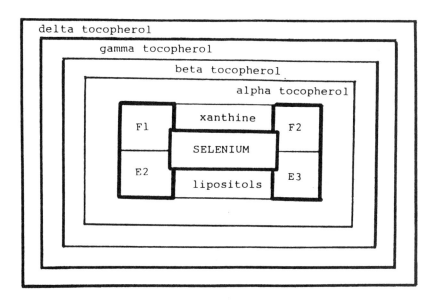

THE FUNCTIONAL ARCHITECTURE OF THE VITAMIN E COMPLEX

Reprinted with permission from Judith DeCava

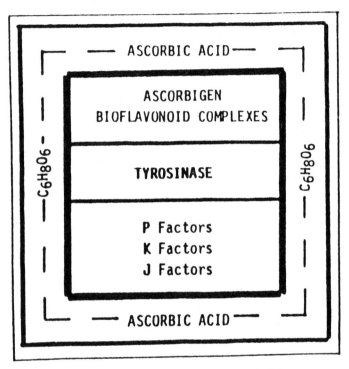

THE FUNCTIONAL ARCHITECTURE
OF VITAMIN C COMPLEX

Reprinted with permission from Judith DeCava

With foods and food concentrates—
containing whole nutritional complexes—
the body can choose its needs for
assimilation and excrete what it does not
need; this is called 'selective absorption'.
On the other hand, with fractionated or
isolated and/or synthetic vitamins, there is
no choice; the body must handle the
chemical in some manner and can suffer
consequences of bio-chemical imbalances
and toxic overdose. (34)

This living vitamin complex can not be taken apart and re-assembled and work the way it did before. In fact, it won't work at all, yet this is exactly what has been done to produce chemically-pure, fractionated vitamins!

Once the vitamin complex has been separated into its components and is dead and inert, it is then that the "scientific method" takes it and develops trials or experiments with it.

Synthetic, fractionated, crystalline-pure
vitamins are not whole, natural
compounds. They are not food which
human systems are familiar with. **How
could any scientist say that the body
does not know the difference between
natural and synthetic vitamins?** (35)

...true science is now judged on the basis
of an experimental method which
measures, classifies, and duplicates

reactions and effects of single chemicals. This rules out testing natural vitamin complexes....This also rules out clinical observation— seeing how a patient is doing and communicating with him/her as to individual benefits, needs, and responses. (36)

Indeed, FDA officials 'have consistently tended to leave out of their thinking both the **human element** in disease and the idea that **cellular malnutrition** is a prominent cause of disease.' (37)

Rats and the RDA's (Recommended Daily Allowances)

The "scientific studies" I have previously mentioned substitute synthetic, crystalline-pure vitamins for whole food complexes, and ignore the human element by substituting rats, chicks, and rabbits for humans. A zoo would *never* feed all the different animals the same food or the same proportions, yet the RDA for humans is now based on **Rat Bioassay.**

The bioassay method is based upon the direct measurement of a vitamin's biological activity in preventing or curing certain specific pathological (disease) conditions in a predetermined experimental animal....This method expresses measurement, in terms of units. So, the amount found to alleviate disease in the rat or other laboratory animal is "translated" into the amount and form needed for humans. (38)

Rats are scavengers. Humans are not. The very physiological makeup of lower animals enables them to eat, digest, and utilize foods and rubbish which we can not. And here is the kicker:

> ...laboratory animals fed ascorbic acid—the manufactured, chemically-pure fraction of the Vitamin C complex— can convert that chemical into the required Vitamin C complex. Such animals with scurvy, when fed ascorbic acid, may improve so that symptoms are relieved. Humans with scurvy, when fed ascorbic acid, **do not improve very much, if at all.** (39)

Getting to the Core of the Matter

Now we come to the reason why synthetic vitamins are *not* good for you. Take, for example, ascorbic acid as Vitamin C. If a person has sufficient reserves of the other components of the C complex (enzymes, coenzymes, antioxidants, trace element activators, and other unknown factors) to recombine and process an intake of ascorbic acid, then that person will experience some improvement for a time. When these reserves are drained, **the ascorbic acid will no longer benefit that person.** The very symptoms that the person was trying to eliminate will return, and the person will then have a full-blown Vitamin C deficiency.

> **This is what occurs with all synthetic vitamins: the body treats them as toxins,** leading to the 'expensive urine' of excess vitamin intake referred to frequently, since the human system via the urinary tract attempts to rid itself of the major quantity of such foreign chemicals. (40)

Many people feel an energy increase, often a euphoria, when they start to take synthetic vitamins. But taking excessive amounts for an extended period of time will cause the effects to reverse. Take, for example, synthetic Thiamine (B1). It "will initially allay fatigue but will eventually **cause** fatigue by the buildup of pyruvic acid. This leads to the vicious cycle of thinking more and more Thiamine is needed, resulting in more and more fatigue along with other accumulated complaints." (41)

Because of the different amounts of stored reserves people have, there are two situations that sincere nutritionists in whole complex research keep pointing out:

1) **Vitamins cannot be standardized, because there is no way of telling what different people's needs are and there is no way to calculate their reserves.**

2) **Individual people's abilities to process, recombine, and eliminate synthetic**

vitamins are full of contradictory effects
(i.e., good, bad, or indifferent effects).

Whole, Natural Vitamins vs. Synthetic

Judith DeCava said it succintly when she said,

…taking one or more such vitamin parts
can create an *imbalance* of vitamins,
which is worse than a *deficiency*. (42)

**Synthetic supplements can unbalance a
person's biochemistry.** (43)

DeCava goes into different studies comparing
whole, natural vs. synthetic vitamins, and the whole,
natural ones always come up ahead. But, do we, as
consumers, know what is natural and what is not? If
the labeling of "natural" is so subjective and undefined,
how can one tell the difference?

The named source of the vitamin is **the best clue.**
So, for your information, the following is a list of the
most common synthetic forms of vitamins. Please take
this book and fold it over and compare this list to the
vitamins and foods you have in your kitchen cupboards.

*You can read more about synthetic vitamins and
their history in my next book, The Biggest Cover-up of
the 20th Century.*

Vitamin	Synthetic Vitamin
Vitamin A	Acetate
	Retinal Palmitate
	Beta Carotene
Vitamin B1	Thiamine HCL
	Thiamine Mononitrate
Vitamin B3	Niacin
Vitamin C	Ascorbic Acid
	Pycnogenols
Vitamin D	Irradiated Ergosterol
Vitamin E	d-Alpha Tocopherol
	dl-Alpha Tocopherol
	d-Alpha Succinate
Vitamin K	K3 or Menadione

We are also used to seeing listings in high milligram potency, however, **a high number of milligrams is also an indication of a synthetic source.**

The B vitamins should be taken as a whole, *with all members of the group.* In nature, all the B's are always found together— never is one isolated from the rest.

Dr. Royal Lee said that a "a natural combination of Vitamin B Complex, a complete source in natural balance including intact synergists, **is from 10 to 50 times more potent in humans, unit for unit,** than is a chemically purified or synthetic complex." Dr. Lee also stressed that in order to get the highest potency and effectiveness, "a number of therapeutically active sources must be tapped", as in Standard Process's Cataplex B (Cataplex means Whole Food Complex).

Standard Process lists on its Cataplex B the following milligrams per 3 tablets:

Thiamine. 0.95mg

Niacin 20.44mg

Vitamin B6 . . . . . . 0.95mg

This is a far cry from the majority of B complexes on the market, which range from 50–100mg for each B.

Cataplex B does not list every B however. Reading the ingredients, the first 2 are Bovine Liver Powder and Nutritional Yeast. So, foods that contain the entire B complex are the base for this product.

Potency Is Not Milligrams or Micrograms

Potency is defined as "the strength, ability, or capacity to bring about a particular result." (44) Potency is taken then to mean effectiveness to the general public. "High Potency" vitamins require a large amount of the fractured vitamin to achieve a specific reaction, although not necessarily a **nutritional** reaction.

A minute amount of a vitamin in its whole food form is more effective nutritionally than a large amount of a synthetic one.

Let us take a look at a story about a medical doctor held captive in a North Korean prisoner of war camp during The Korean War (1950–1953).

After a period of time with an inadequate diet, many of the doctor's fellow prisoners of war began to show signs of beriberi, a disease that results from a severe thiamin (B1) deficiency. He notified The Red

Cross, and they sent him some B1, in the synthetic form, Thiamine HCL. The doctor gave this to his patients, but their health continued to deteriorate. This puzzled him, since B1 was the medical treatment recommended in the <u>Materia Medica</u>.

The doctor's North Korean guards whispered to him that the beriberi could be cured by using rice polish, the nutritive-rich germ of the rice that is removed when rice is refined. He thought it was absurd, but he had nothing to lose, so he started giving his patients a **teaspoon or more of rice polish everyday.** Within a short time, his patients symptoms started to abate and the beriberi plague ceased!

It is important to note here that it would take a ton (2,000 pounds) of unmilled rice to produce a level teaspoon of thiamin (B1)!!! **The amount the prisoners of war were getting would equate down to the amount on the head of pin!**

Synthetics Are Not as Effective

Vitamin E "loses up to *99%* of its potency when seperated from its natural synergists." (45) When you take just the tocopherols, you are throwing out the real Vitamin E. The tocopherols are nature's way of protecting and preserving Vitamin E, like the peel of a banana.

> In one test study, the vitamin E-deficient laboratory animals fed tocopherols died *sooner* then the control animals that received no vitamin at all. (46)

Silver foxes were fed a synthetic diet so that every component of the diet would be known. The animals were given all of the known B vitamins — in synthetic form — but they did not grow; their fur deteriorated, and finally they died. Another group of foxes on the same diet were given a change after a short time: added to their rations was yeast and liver, both sources of natural whole B complex. These animals grew normally and the quality of their fur improved with their health. (47)

Modern-day studies, utilizing ascorbic acid (the crystalline-pure fraction) rather than vitamin C complex, find the synthetic fraction has virtually no effect on pneumonia, bronchitis, or other pulmonary problems even though sufferers show low serum levels of vitamin C…daily intake of ascorbic acid supplements reduces the total white blood cell count, compromising the immune response rather than assisting it. (48)

Confusion around ascorbic acid is created by reports of how it has helped to fight colds and infections. Dr. Jensen points out that "the answer probably lies more in ascorbic acid's pH balance influence (Acid/Alkaline balance) than any other factor." (49) Since most infectious bacteria thrive in an alkaline pH, high consumption of ascorbic acid then creates an acid environment that the bacteria cannot thrive in. Dr. D.C. Jarvis, in his book Folk Medicine, talks about the importance of the Acid/Alkaline balance in the body's immune system. Jarvis promotes the intake of 2–3 tablespoons of apple cider vinegar daily. Apple cider vinegar is 5% *acetic acid*, which is normally found in the body.

Over and over again, it has been proven that the natural, whole food complexes that Mother Nature created are perfectly balanced to work with human physiology to correct a vast number of disorders. However, it is to be emphasized here that a good diet is the basis of health, and ***supplements are the means of catching up for lost time nutritionally.***

Antioxidants—The Controversy

The controversy over the need for antioxidants has been going on for some time. Those who advocate the need for antioxidants usually know nothing about whole food complexes. Remember, most of the news on vitamins from 1962 onward has been "nearly or entirely all based on studies using the fractionated, crystalline-pure, synthetic chemicals." (50)

Antioxidants are the part of the vitamin complex that prevent or inhibit oxidation. Vitamin E is a natural part of polyunsaturated fatty acids and protects oils from deteriorating. In fact, if the oil is rancid, it indicates that the Vitamin E, A, and carotenes have been destroyed. And, **Vitamin E (Alpha tocopherols), Vitamin C (ascorbic acid), and Beta carotene are the most widely touted antioxidants.**

Using antioxidants alone as nutritional supplements means ingesting fractions, isolated substances, not whole complexes. **It would be like eating the peel of a banana without the banana, or like eating the shell of a nut without the nut meat.** (51)

To make matters worse, most commercial antioxidants are produced in pharmaceutical manufacturing plants. "Hoffman-LaRouche, for example, a huge pharmaceutical (drug) conglomerate, is building a plant in Freeport, Texas, to turn out **350 tons of synthetic beta-carotene,** or enough to supply a six milligram capsule daily to every American adult every year." (52)

This crystalline-pure form cannot perform as a nutrient. To attribute the beneficial effects of fruits and vegetables to a single food component, such as carotenes, is useless. There are 50 to 60 carotenes found in the typical American diet, and "humans need complex food sources of even similar or related nutrients, this according to individual needs at specific times." (53)

We hear much talk about **"free radicals"** attacking human cells and weakening our immune systems. Oxidation is a process whereby a molecule contains one or more unpaired electrons (Atoms contain a nucleus, protons, neutrons, and electrons. The electrons move around the nucleus in pairs.). In the free radical *theory,* these molecules try to pick up an electron from another molecule, thus starting a chain reaction.

However, as Judith DeCava's studies point out, most honest scientists know that "every compound excreted by the body is in one form or another bound to oxygen for elimination." (54) In simple terms, oxidation is nature's way of dealing with tissues that are injured by removing damaged cells. It is also a normal way to eliminate cellular waste and debris.

Antioxidants as a Fad

Most of the research on synthesized antioxidants has been done in test tubes or on microscopic slides, with little concern about *the human body's ability to absorb them.* With a vast majority of studies not performed on humans, how can anyone promote unknown benefits?

In fact, too many synthetic antioxidants can cause fatigue and muscle weakness. Denham Harman, M.D., Ph.D., the "father" of the free radical theory of aging, said that he personally would take more antioxidants, but "I can't afford to be fatigued." (55) What he listed as his personal intake was **400iu of "Vitamin E", 2,000mg of "Vitamin C", and 25,000iu of Beta-carotene every day.**

Toxic effects from large intakes of synthetic antioxidants have been reported, which are a scary effect from supplements that are supposed to prevent disease and aging. Natural food complexes *do not* cause adverse effects.

So, antioxidants are widely touted for all of us to take, *yet:*

1) The process, oxidation, that synthetic antioxidants are supposed to protect us from, is a natural by-product of cellular combustion.

2) When taken in large doses, these synthetic antioxidants cause fatigue and muscular weakness.

3) When taken in even larger doses, these synthetic antioxidants are *toxic.*

Here is a prime example of a "new medical fact" that has become an accepted way of thinking for nutritionally-minded people. If this is not a *fad,* what is?

Fads, Trends, and Bold-Faced Lies

Fad is defined by Webster as, "an exaggeratedly fussy attitude, especially about eating or not eating certain kinds of food." My definition of a "Fad" is:

1) You keep eating a certain way, even though you look and feel worse.

2) You keep eating a certain way, because it is advertised and talked about, even though you look and feel worse.

3) You know all of the "scientific reasons" for eating this way, even though you look and feel worse.

All of these definitions certainly fit into our times today. People keep eating low-fat in spite of the obesity, heart disease, and diabetes all around them.

Webster defines a trend as, "a dominant movement revealed by a statistical process". Americans have been on an unnatural trend in their food sources for nearly 100 years. As Dr. Jensen and Mark Anderson in <u>Empty Harvest</u> put it, **"As a culture, we are not just unnatural — it is deeper. We are anti-natural."** (56)

Bold-faced is defined by Webster as, "showing an impudent lack of shame." An impudent lack of shame is evident by those who proclaim that the human body cannot tell the difference between natural and synthetic vitamins and foods.

Why Do I Need Vitamins and Minerals if I'm Eating Well?

Vitamins are factors that cause health. Vitamins act as facilitators in all of the chemical reactions in the body. Because most people have likes and dislikes that keep them from eating foods such as kale, broccoli, etc…in the quantities necessary to get the needed nutrients from them, **vitamin supplements are a must.**

Remember, due to chemical fertilizers which keep plants from absorbing trace minerals and commercial milling of wheat and other grains that remove all nutrients, Americans have been consuming a very poor diet since WWI. These nutritional deficiencies have caused:

> …the previously unanticipated phenomenon of **many genetically transmitted conditions,** because they originated in deficiency and poisoning patterns of forebearers. (57)

> Dr. Lee said in 1950, *'Trace mineral deficiency, it is evident, can act also to*

impair hereditary transmission. As these trace minerals and determinants (cell blueprints) are combined organically into protein linkages, it is evident how the nature of these minerals in our foods are of vital importance.' (58)

The monumental work, <u>Nutrition and Physical Degeneration</u>, by Dr. Weston Price, D.D.S., graphically shows that **inferior genetic traits were passed along to the next generation** as soon as the parents began to eat what Dr. Price called "the foods of commerce".

Dr. Price traveled to primitive cultures around the world in the 1930's and photographed two different groups within each culture. One group ate their traditional, unadulterated diet. The second group ate civilized counterfeit and adulterated foods. (See the photographs on the next 3 pages)

So, basically *we are the second, third, and fourth generations in this synthetic diet transmission. We are in need of as much nutritional building as we can possibly get.* To continue to consume synthetic vitamins to build up an immune system already weakened by synthetic foods and vitamins will not work!

In fact, these synthetic vitamins are often poisonous. "In January of 1952, Dr. Lee announced: 'I could write volumes on how synthetic vitamins like thiamine castrate the descendants of the victim who uses even as much as double the daily requirement.'" (80) Dr. Lee then cited a study by Dr. Barnett Sure (Jol. Natr., Aug., 1939). Dr. Sure studied two groups of pigs, feeding one group twice the daily requirement of synthetic B and the other group the same amount of

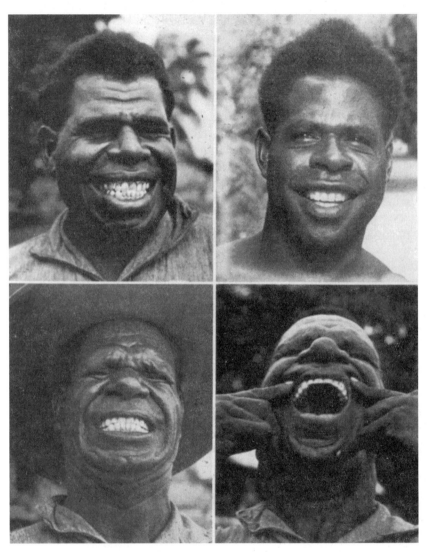

Photos and captions by permission of the Price-Pottenger Foundation, California.

Natives on the islands of the Great Barrier Reef. The dental arches here reach a high degree of excellence.

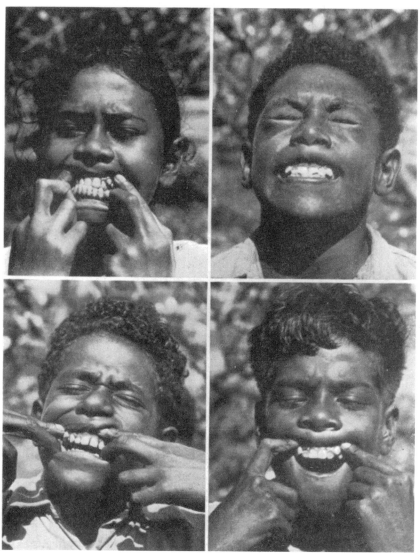

The contrast between the primitive and modernized natives in facial and dental arch form is as striking here as elsewhere. These young natives were born to parents who had adopted our modern foods of commerce. Note the narrowed faces and dental arches with pinched nostrils and crowding of the teeth. Their magnificent heredity could not protect them.

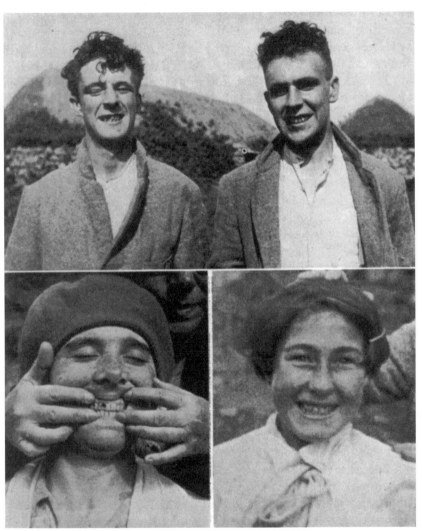

Photos and captions by permission of the Price-Pottenger Foundation, California.

Above: brothers, Isle of Harris. The younger at left uses modern food and has rampant tooth decay. Brother at right uses native food and has excellent teeth. Note narrowed face and arch of younger brother. Below: typical rampant tooth decay, modernized Gaelic. Right: typical excellent teeth of primitive Gaelic.

natural B. "The result: **ALL** of the first generation offspring from the pigs fed the synthetic vitamin were **STERILE.**" (81) It is obvious that synthetic B, in addition to NOT being a nutrient, is a genetic poison.

Humans, unlike pigs, take more than one generation to reap this genetic damage. A 1981 report from The University of Florida stated that the American male sperm count in 1929 was at approximately 100 million sperm cells per milliliter of semen. By 1973 the sperm count had dropped to 60 million/ml. Then seven years later, in 1980, **the average count had dropped to 20 million/ml.!**

> What in the world happened to bring about such a horrible drop in male fertility in just 61 years? One very possible explanation could very well lie in the historical use of synthetic B and other counterfeit nutrients.... Since World War II the American people, and people of other countries as well, have had a daily ration of a genetic poison in most of the bread, flour products, cereals and other food items that are forced, by law, to enrich with the only cost-feasible enricher: *synthetic vitamins.* (82)

A Word About Standard Process

Most Americans have never heard of Dr. Royal Lee, and his name should be a household word. As previously mentioned, Dr. Lee was a brilliant and prolific electronic inventor, with more than 100 electrical patents. From the 1920's to the mid-1960's, Dr. Lee amassed information about plant, animal, and human health and how it all tied into the soil, food processing, diet, and nutrition.

With this information, he founded The Lee Foundation for Nutritional Research, a clearing house of information for doctors, lay people, and farmers. In 1929, he formulated *Catalyn,* a concentrated multiple vitamin, trace mineral, and enzyme product. Every time a new trace mineral, enzyme, or micro-nutrient is discovered, **Catalyn is analyzed, and the substance is always found to be present in it.**

Dr. Lee once said that it took him longer to develop a nutritional formula than to come up with one of his electrical inventions. This was due to the complexity of factors already present in nature.

As doctors would encounter some illness or disease in the field, Dr. Lee would go to his laboratory and develop a *whole food supplement* that would support a natural healing process. Thus, the entire Standard Process line came into being.

Because Dr. Lee insisted that foods were therapeutic, he was always in court, fighting the FDA which insisted that only drugs could be called therapeutic. Finally, he was told to either burn every copy of his Therapeutic Food Manual, or go to jail for 7 years!!! He was willing to go, but his family begged him not to, so all of the manuals were burned! Remember what the German chemical industrialists did to Julius Hensel's book on rock dust. Hensel's book could not be found for many years, and was squelched so that the consumers were lead to conclude that it was false. Fortunately for us, a copy of Dr. Lee's book was stored in the archives of a non-profit organization and reprinted years later for the benefit of all.

Standard Process whole food supplements are made according to the rigid guidelines set by Dr. Lee. All of the natural foods used are grown on rich farmland, in thick, black topsoil that is free from chemical fertilizers and pesticides. Dr. Lee's formulas are made from **whole foods concentrated to clinical potency.** For example, Standard Process takes **3,000** gallons of beets and concentrates them into a powder that could fit into a briefcase. This is then added to Standard Process' Betafood and AF Betafood, which help the gall bladder.

With Standard Process' **Cataplex E** (Cataplex means whole complex), you get the E complex in the form that Dr. Lee discovered was the richest source of the E complex: **the juice of the whole pea plant!**

If this sounds weak or impotent, remember what potency really is: *The strength, ability, or capacity to bring about a particular result.*

These potent nutrients can help us to catch up for lost time nutritionally. What this catching up for lost time nutritionally really means is best illustrated by the following quote from Dr. Bruce West.

> If you had a heart problem with high blood fats and poor digestion, my best R_x would be some powerful dietary changes. For starters, if this were feasible, I would like to see you consume daily: a pound of raw, organic liver; a couple buckets of organic wheat germ and high-selenium yeast; a

small wheelbarrow full of organic beets and beet tops; gallons of freshly squeezed vegetable juices; and plenty of raw, fresh-pressed organic oils such as flax oil.

Naturally, this is impossible. So, instead we use supplements which are *condensed from these foods and other nutrients.* (85)

Since Dr. Lee believed that we, as humans, need the nutrition from both plants and animals, many Standard Process products have both. An example of this would be Folic acid and B12. Folic acid is derived from plants, B12 from liver. So Standard Process has Carrot Powder and Bovine Liver as their listed sources for these vitamins. All Standard Process products are tested and retested countless times by Certified Lab Techs to ensure the *purity* of all nutrients used.

The Work in Nutrition Has Already Been Done!

Everything we need to know about nutrition has already been done by Mother Nature herself. Nature is the chemist, and all that a biochemist can do is to unlock the *already existing relationships* within and between all of these micronutrient factors, split them up, identify them, and test them to see what happens if a laboratory animal goes without them.

This happens on a regular basis. Everyday a "new" discovery hits the news media. (Co Enzyme Q-10, Co Enzyme PQQ, Antioxidants, Selenium, Pycnogenols, Phyto-chemicals, etc...)

The interesting thing here is that Standard Process contains all of these "new" discoveries, because whole food supplements contain all of the synergists (enzymes, coenzymes, trace minerals, and all of the **unknown** factors yet to be discovered). By taking foods intact, you always get everything you need. You also do not have to play the guessing game of figuring out how much of a new discovery you need to take.

When you have a bottle of Vitamin E (d-Alpha tocopherol), a bottle of selenium, and a bottle of Co-enzyme Q-10, what you actually have are parts of the E complex that are being purchased separately. It takes some playing around to get the dosages right, but most importantly, *what you are getting is dead and inert, and there are many other components which you are not getting.*

A Sobering Word

J.I. Rodale, the American naturalist, wrote wisely in his classic work The Complete Book of Food and Nutrition:

> We **must** take vitamins if we wish to be
> healthy and the nation as a whole must do
> it, or God alone knows what will happen
> to the second or third generations coming
> up—generations inheriting weaknesses
> passed on to them by us, generations
> which few of us will live to see unless we
> augment our diet with vitamins and
> minerals. And, as parting advice, don't

take coal tar (synthetic) vitamins.
Examine every bottle. Be sure that the vitamins you take are extracted from food. Scientific research proves that this is best. (59)

It couldn't have been said any better. Remember, Thiamine HCL and Thiamine Mononitrate come from coal tar *and are in all commercial breads.* Vitamin B12 comes from activated sewage sludge and vitamin D is concocted from irradiated oil.

Ancient Civilizations and Low Fat Diets

With our food supply polluted and our synthetic vitamins in hand, what else can be done to ruin our health? Well, we could be encouraged to eat a diet low in fats and protein and high in carbohydrates, thus insuring that we ingest *more refined, chemicalized foods and create blood sugar problems* that really do us in.

Let's go back in time, with Drs. Mary and Michael Eades, whose book, <u>Protein Power</u>, was published in January, 1996. The Eades start with the fact that "for 2 million years humans ate a diet of mainly meat, fat, nuts, and berries. 8,000 years ago we learned to farm, and as our consumption of grain increased, our health declined. That is only 400 to 500 generations ago, whereas genetic evolutionary changes take a minimum of 1,000 generations— or **another** 8,000 to 10,000 years." (60)

In fact, the Drs. Eades note that anthropologists can tell whether the skull they are examining was that of a hunter-gatherer (protein eater) or a farmer (mainly carbohydrate eater). The well-formed, strong bones and teeth belong to the tall hunters. The farmers have signs of stunted growth and tooth decay.

Since there is so much information available to us about the ancient Egyptians, through their records and their mummies, they are a good starting point for historical nutritional evaluation. **We know that they ate the perfect low-fat diet: lots of whole grains, fresh fruits and vegetables, along with some fish and fowl, and hardly any fat.**

So what do paleopathologists find when they examine these mummies? (Paleopathology, among other modern techniques, applies forensic science to the early remains of man) They can tell what the corpse died of, its age, sex, health status, and numerous other things.

When paleopathologists dissected the arteries of the Egyptian mummies, they did not find smooth, supple arterial walls but rather **arteries choked with greasy, cholesterol-laden deposits** that were often calcified, exhibiting an advanced stage of atherosclerotic disease. Many subjects had arteries that were scarred and thickened, indicating the presence of high blood pressure. Pathologists today find the same diseased changes when examining tissue from a victim of heart attack, stroke, diabetes, or other disease found in conjunction with late-stage heart disease. In fact **it appears that cardiovascular**

disease was as prevalent in ancient Egypt as it is in America today. (61)

What's Happening Here?

Since humans were hunter-gatherers for such a long period, our metabolisms were designed to cope with food supplies that were unpredictable. What enabled us to store food for the lean times was *insulin.*

> Unfortunately, a diet heavy in carbohydrate also sends our insulin levels soaring, and our body interprets this as a need to store calories, to make cholesterol, and to conserve water— all important to our survival way back then. (62)

We would constantly have to be hooked up to our energy source (food) in order to merely function, if it were not for insulin. Insulin stores fat in our bodies, and this fat acts like a built-in battery, which gets re-charged when we eat, and used for energy when we don't.

So, diet is the best way to control insulin, in fact, it is the *only* way. **Consumption of large quantities of carbohydrate produce large quantities of insulin.** This is because carbohydrates are composed of various sugar molecules, or glucose, bonded chemically. Once you have eaten a carbohydrate, even a *complex* carbohydrate, your body has digestive enzymes that break these chemical bonds and release the sugar molecules into the blood.

Insulin springs into action when the blood sugar starts to climb too high, as it does after a carbohydrate meal. The elevated blood sugar triggers the pancreas to synthesize and release insulin into the bloodstream. This insulin first makes a pass through the liver, where it shuts down any sugar production that may still be going on, then travels on to the rest of the body, where it acts on sensors or receptors scattered across the surfaces of muscle and fat cells. These receptors, when activated by insulin, initiate a series of reactions that pump sugar (along with protein and fat) from the blood into the interior of the cells for use now or storage for later. Insulin stimulates the fat cells to take up fat and sugar from the blood and store it away as body fat, especially in the middle of the body, within the abdomen, and around the vital organs. (63)

Which Way is Your Metabolism Going?

Since nature over and over again works with complementary factors (witness the fungus-bacteria relationship in plants), it is no wonder that our bodies have two hormones, *insulin* and *glucagon*, to store and release energy. **Insulin causes our metabolism to store excess food energy for later and keeps our blood sugar from getting too high. Glucagon allows our bodies to burn our stored fat for energy and keeps our blood sugar from getting too low.**

These functions of storing fat or burning fat are active to some degree all the time. The question is, which energy pathway predominates? **Are we mainly storing or mainly burning fat for energy?** It is important to note that the fat in the bloodstream could come from these sources:

1) **fat consumed in the diet**

2) **fat made from excess carbohydrate and protein in the diet**

3) **fat liberated from storage in the fat cells**

So, our bodies can make plenty of fat from carbohydrate—low fat cookies and potato chips included!

In fact, **the number-one foods consumed by most Americans** are white bread, rolls, and crackers. Number-two are doughnuts, cookies, and cake, and number-three are alcoholic beverages. (Statistics from a survey conducted in 1983 by the National Center for Health Statisitics)

The Drs. Eades point out that *the combination of high carbohydrate with low protein caused the greatest increase in insulin production- more than carbohydrate itself.* This is interesting, especially in light of the foods Americans love, like hamburgers and fries, pizza, macaroni and cheese, eggs and hash browns, cereal and milk, etc…, all protein/carbohydrate combinations. The Drs. Eades also note that dietary fat in and of itself cannot cause problems with cholesterol unless you eat carbohydrates with the fat.

Dieting is Failing

In a brilliant and controversial essay on intelligence published in the winter 1969 issue of *Harvard Educational Review,* Arthur R. Jensen, a professor of psychology at the University of California at Berkeley, wrote: 'In other fields, when bridges do not stand, when aircraft do not fly, when machines do not work, when treatments do not cure, despite all conscientious efforts on the part of many persons to make them do so, **one begins to question the basic assumptions, principles, theories, and hypotheses** that guide one's efforts.' Most physicians, dieticians, and nutritionists have been locked in the notorious clean and well-lit prison of a single idea for decades. These experts have been treating obesity with low-calorie, low-fat, high-complex-carbohydrate diets, then standing around wringing their hands, watching 95% of their patients regain their weight. Perhaps inevitably they blame the patient for the failure. (64)

Obviously, the low-fat, high-carbohydrate diet is out of step with people's biochemistry— in fact, it actually strengthens an enzyme called *Lipoprotein Lipase*—a fat storage enzyme. To switch to a high-protein, low-carbohydrate diet keeps insulin levels low, so that the Lipoprotein Lipase is not getting ***any*** stimulation. Instead, *Hormone-Sensitive Lipase,* which releases fat from the fat cells into the blood, is stimulated.

More Than Just Fat

High insulin levels are the major cause of obesity, but according to Drs. Eades and the many medical studies they quote, the following are all symptoms of elevated insulin levels:

1) **High Blood Pressure**

2) **High Blood Cholesterol and Triglyceride Levels**

3) **Diabetes (Adult-onset specifically)**

4) **Heart Disease**

High Blood Pressure

Excessive insulin causes high blood pressure by forcing the kidneys to retain sodium, even when there is too much, and this results in fluid retention. In another way, excessive insulin increases the thickness of the arterial walls, making them less elastic and narrower. In a final way, insulin stimulates the adrenals to constrict the blood vessels and increase the heart rate, thus raising blood pressure.

Unfortunately, most doctors treat only the symptoms and often in a way that makes the real problem worse. If, for example, you go to your doctor and find that your cholesterol level and blood pressure are too high, we can just about guarantee that you will leave the office with instructions to go on a low-fat diet and to return to the office for a recheck in a month or so. If you follow this advice and go on the low-fat diet, what happens? By decreasing your fat intake you usually decrease your protein intake, because virtually all foods that are protein-rich contain substantial amounts of fat. Meat, eggs, cheese, most dairy products—the best sources of complete dietary protein— are all taboo or severely restricted on a low-fat diet. With this protein and fat restriction, the only food component left in the diet is carbohydrate, which by default results in your eating a high-carbohydrate, low-protein diet—the very diet that maximizes insulin production. If you had hyperinsulinemia to begin with— and if you have elevated cholesterol and high blood pressure, you can bet that you do— increasing your body's production of insulin isn't going to help. A month later, your doctor will probably find that your cholesterol has decreased slightly (due to the caloric restriction), but not enough to put it in the normal range, and that your blood pressure is about the same, maybe even a little higher. Now when you leave the office, you'll go with a prescription for a high blood pressure medicine, a more stringent diet, and perhaps a prescription for a cholesterol-lowering medicine as well.

You leave with your prescriptions, your sample medicines, your new diet instruction sheets, and a nagging worry. You know that you followed the diet to the letter, so why didn't it work? And you wonder, am I going to have to take these medicines for the rest of my life? You comply with your doctor's orders and return at the appointed time for your follow-up visit. Your doctor finds that your blood pressure is down to normal and your cholesterol level has fallen into the normal range. You are relieved, and this time when you leave you're happy, your doctor ishappy, and the drug companies are ecstatic: they have just signed you on as a new customer to the tune of between $50 and $200 per month for life.

On the surface this story seems to have a happy ending, but does it really? While looking for all the world like another triumph of modern medicine over disease, the treatment of your elevated cholesterol and high blood pressure is only a camouflage. (65)

WARNING: The Drs. Eades found that a high protein/low carbohydrate diet was so effective in lowering blood pressure that their patients who were on medication to lower their blood pressure felt dizzy and faint within a few days, and had to be taken off of their medication very quickly. So, do not attempt this diet if you are on medication to lower your blood pressure without being under the care of a physician.

Enter Cholesterol

At the beginning of their chapter in <u>Protein Power</u> entitled "Cholesterol Madness," the Drs. Eades let you know that, with careful reading, "by the time you finish this chapter you will know more about cholesterol than 95 per cent of the physicians in practice today." (86)

And, of course, cholesterol has become big business. **Whenever mass paranoia starts to brew, a legion rises up ready to exploit it.** The food processing industry and their advertisers now emblazon the containers of edibles as diverse as soft drinks and cornflakes with the superfluous statement 'contains no cholesterol'. Cholesterol angst is not lost on the various governmental and private research funding bodies responsible for underwriting all kinds of medical research. These groups disburse hundreds of millions of dollars to eager research labs throughout the world, allowing them to pursue the secrets of cholesterol in ever-more-intricate studies. (66)

Cholesterol, as the Drs. Eades point out, is essential for life. Only 7% of the body's cholesterol is found in the blood. "The bulk of the cholesterol in your body, the other 93%, is located in every cell of the body, where its unique waxy, soapy consistency provides the cell membranes with their structural integrity and regulates the flow of nutrients into and waste products out of the cells." (67) Some cholesterol comes from food, but 80% is produced by the body itself, mostly in the liver.

Cholesterol is the building block for hormones and the major component of liver bile, and your brain and nerves need cholesterol for normal electrical signal transmission.

The number one point to remember here is that the **cholesterol levels are regulated *inside* the cell.** When the supply runs low, the cell can either make more cholesterol or send LDL receptors (messengers) to the surface and snatch the next circulating LDL particle out of the blood.

LDL (Low Density Lipoprotein) is sometimes seen as the villain in the cholesterol drama. And it can be, if there is too much of it. But the truth is, there is again a natural relationship between LDL and HDL (High Density Lipoprotein). LDL carries cholesterol to the tissues for deposition and HDL gathers cholesterol from these tissues and carries it back to the liver to be disposed of. The flow one way or the other is what medical researchers have used to quantify risk for heart disease.

Insulin cranks up the cell's cholesterol-manufacturing ability, so that they don't need to snatch any from the bloodstream and LDL levels rise. Clearly, the more LDL receptors we have pulling cholesterol from the blood, the better.

The artery-clogging damage that occurs with elevated insulin levels is analogous to "having a big powerful air conditioner in a house and putting the thermostat that controls it into a small, hot, airtight closet. The cooling machinery could be cranking out enough cold air to form icicles on the woodwork throughout the house, but the thermostat in the closet would never know. As far as it knows, the air is hot and needs cooling, so it calls for more cold air, and in spite of the icicles forming on it, the air conditioner keeps huffing and struggling along to pump cold air out." (68) So, the cholesterol plaque is like the icicles in the house.

> The key to lowering elevated cholesterol levels is not in the restriction of dietary cholesterol or fat but in the dietary manipulation of the internal cholesterol regulatory system. (69)

> ...By eating a diet that reduces insulin levels...you reduce the signal telling the cells to make cholesterol, they *must* harvest it from the blood to have enough, and your blood cholesterol levels— especially the "bad" LDL—fall rapidly. Even while eating a diet that contains red meat, egg yolk, cheese, butter, and cream,

as long as you control your insulin output, your cholesterol will remain in the healthy 180–200 mg/dl range. (87)

Diabetes

In the case of Type II or Adult Onset Diabetes, a stage called "insulin resistance" or "impaired glucose tolerance" is a forerunner. Years of lifestyle abuse start in childhood. Studies done in the United States have shown that many children from ages five on consume approximately one cup (200 grams) of sugar a day. If you included the carbohydrate they consume, that figure would double. (Remember, **any carbohydrate is metabolized exactly like sugar**)

After 30 or 40 years of this excess, the metabolic gears start to slip and **middle age spread sets in.** The person may even be eating less, but he/she is gaining weight. The insulin sensors in the tissues become more and more sluggish, and the pancreatic beta cells start working overtime to make more and more insulin to bring the blood sugar back into the normal range. At this point, if the blood glucose exceeds a certain threshold, typically 140 mg/dl, it will then be at such a high concentration in the blood that it destroys the beta cells.

This increase in blood sugar, in addition to going through the stage of insulin resistance to diabetes, has emotional components as well as physical. The "enriched" grains that most people consume cause vitamin depletion, especially the B complex. Some of the symptoms of B Complex Deficiency Syndrome, as it is called, are fatigue, nervousness, depression, and forgetfullness.

Also, there is an entire body of work (which will not be gotten into here) that addresses the lack of amino acids as being an important component in clinically depressed individuals.

The important thing to remember here is that *diet is the only method available to treat excess insulin.* A high-protein, low-carbohydrate diet can reduce insulin levels in a matter of days and reduce blood pressure and cholesterol or triglyceride levels. In a period of months, it can result in a steady loss of excess stored body fat.

> It's important to remember, however, that even though the regimen works rapidly to return insulin sensitivity to normal in most people, it works only as long as you follow it. It doesn't return you to your childhood levels of imperviousness to carbohydrate assault. You must continue to follow the guidelines to maintain the changes; a return to your former eating habits will return you to your former problems. (70)

Heart Disease

In the case of heart disease, problems arise when the flow of blood to any area of the heart is reduced significantly, or is cut off completely. Apparently, **the heart could pump on forever with adequate supplies of oxygen-rich blood.**

When a person has a heart attack, it is usually brought on by a blockage of a coronary artery created by the build-up of plaque.

> Plaque forms over a long period of time, progressing in a stepwise fashion, starting with the infiltration of cholesterol into the lining of the artery and proceeding to the development of the mature lesion. (71)

> The five steps in the plaque-forming process are:

1) **Cholesterol in the LDL form makes its way into the arterial lining.**

2) **The trapped cholesterol becomes chemically altered.**

3) **Foam cells form. These are scavenger cells that eat the altered LDL and bloat up.**

4) **Fatty streaks form as there are more and more foam cells.**

5) **These fatty streaks collect to form plaque.**

> *Insulin,* by its action on the cholesterol synthesis pathway located within the cells, **helps to create and sustain excess amounts of LDL in blood...** and also increases the proliferation of smooth muscle cells in the artery and their migration into the area of plaque formation. (72)

In a study done in the 1960's by Dr. Anatolio Cruz, insulin was injected into the large arteries in the legs of dogs. One leg was injected with insulin. The other leg was injected with saline. After eight months, the arteries injected with insulin had a pronounced accumulation of cholesterol and were already thickening.

Don't Forget the Eicosanoids

I have mainly used the Drs. Eades' book to illustrate the importance of a high-protein, low-carbohydrate diet. But, <u>Dr. Atkins New Dietary Revolution</u> and Dr. Barry Sears' <u>The Zone</u> are both currently on the New York Times Best Sellers List and both expound the same dietary principles.

It is Dr. Sears who brought eicosanoids into the public arena. He even describes ***optimal health*** as the dynamic balance between the various eicosanoids.

> You can view eicosanoids as the biological glue that holds together the human body. In that regard they are the most powerful agents known to man, yet they are totally controlled by diet.
> *Barry Sears, Ph.D.,* author of <u>The Zone</u>

Again, our body works as a balance of opposing forces. ***There are almost 100 powerful eicosanoids in the body.*** They control whether your blood vessels contract or dilate, whether you have a headache or not, inflammation in a joint or not, whether you suffer from allergies or do not, sleep well or poorly, whether you form tumors or not, and on and on. In fact, most cardiac drugs are eicosanoids inhibitors.

So, *there are "good" and "bad" eicosanoids,* and they are all produced from the dietary fat *Linoleic acid,* which is present in practically all foods. Essential fatty acids are the building blocks of eicosanoids, but *Linoleic acid* is the only true essential fat from which all other fats can be made.

The Drs. Eades point out that foods have an influence on the eicosanoid factory at 2 different points:

1) **Where Linoleic acid enters the system.** Since *Linoleic acid* is found in nearly all foods, a person should have plenty available.

2) **Where the critical gatekeeper enzyme *delta 6 desaturase* shifts the production to good or bad eicosanoids.** Dietary protein is the *only* factor that speeds up this gatekeeper. The factors that slow it down are:
   A) **Aging**
   B) **Stress**
   C) **Disease**
   D) **Trans-fatty acids,** such as margarine and the partially-hydrogenated oils found in thousands of commercial foods "cause health damage because they *inhibit* the formation of good eicosanoids." (73)

E) **High-Carbohydrate, Low- Protein Diets** stimulate excess insulin, which sends the production of bad eicosanoids soaring.

Obviously, there is not too much we can do about aging. Our fast-paced American way of life makes stress a common factor in almost everyone's life and no matter how hard we try, we can still get the occasional cold or flu.

Since aging, stress, and disease are pretty much beyond our control, we are left with the remaining three factors, *all dietary.* By excercising control and not consuming trans-fatty acids, adding good oils to our diets, and switching to a high protein, low carbohydrate diet, we can do a lot to produce good eicosanoids and experience good health.

A Doctor's View

From the previous explanations of all of the havoc that excess insulin causes in our bodies, it is no wonder that more and more medical doctors are questioning the very principles on which our health system is based.

Dr. Atkins, in his <u>Health Revelations</u> (Vol. IV, No. 5, May 1996), talks about the rigid orthodoxy of <u>Cecil's Textbook of Medicine</u>, which is the book that gets doctors through medical school. Atkins says that:

"Cecil's teems with…misinformation…the book's common denominator is preservation of an outdated status quo, which can be summed up this way: **'Make sure non-pharmacological treatments fail, then prescribe drugs.'** That rigid teaching is a miseducation and an unconscionable disservice to patients. A doctor who passed the boards because he or she knew everything in Cecil's Textbook of Medicine would have no value at the Atkins Center. Treatment by textbook has no place in your health, either." (74)

The growing frustration with standard medical views is also illustrated in the following:

> Robert D. Willix, Jr., M.D., was a hard-charging medical doctor who had developed the only open-heart surgery program in the state of South Dakota. He performed about 2,000 coronary bypass operations and finally realized he was not helping people. He has not picked up a scalpel since 1981, but, he says, 'I've saved more patients than I did as a surgeon.' Simply, he explains, 'I used to look at things the same way as the medical establishment. Basically, their view is that the body is a sort of machine you fix when it breaks down. I shucked off this dangerous, mistaken point of view and learned how human beings really work. Over the past 40 years, evidence has been piling up that the way the body works is totally different from what the medical profession thinks.' Nevertheless, the

medical way of thinking still prevails. (75)

Even though these standard medical views prevail, it is the Drs. Atkins, Eades, Sears, Willix, and others who are getting their messages out there, and they *need to be heard.*

Digestion vs. Indigestion

Well, by now we are all set to start eating more protein. But, we stop and think: one of the reasons many of us stopped eating meat was that it gave us heartburn. Also, sometimes after eating meat, we felt sluggish and the food just sat in our stomachs.

Indigestion plagues almost everyone. **Tagamet is the #1 selling drug in the world,** and vending machines will soon start carrying Pepsid AC and Tums. "Epigastral reflux" is becoming a household word. So, indigestion is common. But, what exactly is **digestion?**

In order to digest food, stay immune from parasites, *and* avoid getting candida, you *must* have plenty of hydrochloric acid (HCL) in your stomach. This "arch-villain" in all the antacid commercials is *really a good guy.* In fact, your stomach is an acid machine!

When the stomach digests, it churns the food and mixes it with HCL, juices, pepsin, and enzymes. If there is no HCL, the food begins to *rot and ferment.* As it ferments, it then develops *abnormal acids* that are stinging and burning. Your stomach starts churning harder and harder, trying to digest the food in it, and sometimes some of these deviant acids, along with what little HCL remains, gets backed up into the esophagus.

What you really need is more HCL, and to take an antacid at this point makes sure that you have a mass of undigested food in your stomach. What doesn't get digested by your stomach then puts a burden on your liver and pancreas to get the job done, and they can't. Your body then begins to get **toxic and full of poisons from this undigested matter.**

Once again, Mother Nature designed the human body with a digestive assembly line to split open food molecules, break them down into vitamins, minerals, trace elements, fatty acids, amino acids, and enzymes. Then your body eliminates what is not used through the bowel.

With an undigested food mass decaying and travelling through the thirty feet of the gastro-intestinal tract, all kinds of undesirable bacteria and viruses start scavenging this waste. Parasites, which could have been inadvertently swallowed and should have been destroyed by the HCL, are now finding a toxic environment to start living in. *Candida Albicans,* a fungus your body has in place to kill undesirable bacteria (remember the bacteria-fungus relationship in plants), starts to multiply in order to handle the ever larger volume of bacteria.

If this sounds disgusting, it is! The body is starting to break down through *this continuous poisoning.*

If you have a concentration of bacteria living in some organ of the body, you have a staph infection or strep in the throat, for instance, they are there because of unhealthy, devitalized tissue and unprocessed metabolic waste...disease is not the presence of something evil, but rather **the lack of the presence of something essential.** (76)

So, eating correctly is important, and digesting it is just as important! Standard Process makes an excellent HCL supplement, Zypan, which also includes pancreatin and pepsin to help the stomach get the job done.

What is Health?

Sadly, we do not even know how to identify good health anymore.

The World Health Organization defines health as 'a state of complete physical, mental, and social well-being and not merely the absence of disease or infirmity.' (77)

Everyday one sees people with pasty, sallow complexions, either yellow, grey, or sometimes even white. That they have poor blood quality is not even thought of. There is hardly a grocery store, fast food chain, or office you can go into without seeing someone with their wrists immobilized in a brace for carpal-tunnel syndrome. We blame repetitive work for this; never does it occur to us that human ligaments are weakened by **insufficient protein, C complex, and trace minerals.**

Babies are born with all kinds of abnormalities, and we just figure that, statistically, this is the way it is. Many people are obese, yet we never look at all of the carbohydrate they consume. Nibbling on a low-fat cookie is even encouraged! Varicose veins, easy bruising, gums that bleed easily, stretch-marks, popping or cracking of the joints, and slipped discs are just accepted as normal wear and tear on the body. No one would ever think that these are signs of *subclinical scurvy,* a C complex deficiency! Impaired wound healing, hair loss, dry skin, and eczema are accepted as a part of our genetic makeup. However, these are all signs of a *Vitamin F, or fatty-acid, deficiency* (Remember, trans-fatty acids can *cause* Vitamin F deficiencies).

We rationalize all this and more and keep on moving—but *tiredly*. Fatigue has gotten so common that we even have a syndrome devoted to it (Chronic Fatigue Syndrome).

Look in the Mirror

One of the most common nutritional deficiencies in America today is **B Complex Deficiency Syndrome.** Some of the symptoms of BCD are:

Indigestion	Anxiety
Weakness and Fatigue	Depression
Dizziness	Mental Confusion
Forgetfullness	Impaired Intellect
Uneasiness	Hostility
Rage	Craving for Sweets

The tendency to cry for no reason is one of the most common complaints. The second and most classical symptom of BCD is **a constant feeling that something dreadful is about to happen.**

Adelle Davis, in her book, <u>Let's Eat Right To Keep Fit</u>, points out that, when the B vitamins are undersupplied, many changes take place in the tongue.

> As the deficiencies of these vitamins become more severe, clumps of taste buds fuse and grow together, pulling apart from other clumps and thus forming grooves or fissures. The first groove usually forms down the center of the tongue. In a severe B-vitamin deficiency, the tongue may be so cut by grooves and fissures that it looks like a relief map of the Grand Canyon and the surrounding territory or a flank steak run through a tenderizing machine. (78)

People who are in a "brain fog" are often deficient in B vitamins. Also, dim vision in the elderly, and swollen, red eyelids is another B vitamin deficiency (B_2 specifically).

With some of these vitamin deficiencies as guidelines, you can see where many Americans are *starving* for different nutrients. Stop taking all of these deficiency signs for granted and get to your health professional and start getting these deficiencies corrected.

Learn more about how to identify nutritional deficiencies in my next book, <u>The Biggest Cover-up of the 20th Century.</u>

Summing Up

This booklet has been presented in an effort to educate you about natural food and soil, whole food supplements vs. synthetic, and the importance of protein and natural fats in the diet. It is an attempt to *go back to the basics of human health,* because it is in the basic diet of our forefathers that we are truely protected from all this craziness.

So much of our modern living tends to desensitize people and hold them in a lethargic state.

...hollow food grown on empty soil keeps...bodies and minds dull, unproductive in manufacturing the chemical compounds of the brain and endocrine system. To once quote Surgeon General Parran, *'Many well-to-do Americans who can eat what they like are so badly fed as to be physically inferior and mentally dull.'*

Enfeebled as such, in this disconnected life, people actually don't want to know what is happening in reality, so they safely read about unreality in supermarket tabloids and popular magazines, which, no matter how outrageous the stories, require no response or action on their parts. They gulp their sugared pop and nibble their hydrogenated chips, oblivious to the garbage and radiation that infiltrates their water, their air, their soil. Pathetically, their biggest fear is 'losing it all'. Afraid of dying, the fear of truly living is greater.

The feeling seems to be, "There is only so much of the 'good life', not everyone can have it, and I am lucky to have my share. I don't know Mother Earth, but I'll rest my soul in the bosom of Mother General Mills, or Mother Exxon, or Mother Squibb, or Mother Del Monte, or Mother Du Pont, or Mother Safeway." Of course, loyalty to these 'mothers' is as deep as a paycheck or discount coupon. (79)

And then we wonder about the crime rate, problems with our children in school, and social problems of all kinds. It is an unhealthy world we live in. All we can do is start with ourselves. We need to get ourselves and our families healthy first, then our friends, and then work gradually out to our community and so on.

So, instead of running from one new "health discovery" to another and ignoring the way our forefathers ate, embrace it. Remember, over 100 years ago people ate fresh whole foods including plenty of meat, butter, and lard. Go back to the basics. It has been proven to work.

Action Steps to Function Optimally

At this point, it is obvious that you need certain basics. According to the Drs. Eades, they are as follows:

1) **Plenty of protein,** ranging from 60-90 grams/day for women and 80-110 grams/day for men. Be sure that, as much as you can, you eat ***antibiotic and hormone-free*** meat and eggs from chickens that are cage-free. Also, raw milk and raw milk products have the most live enzymes and vitamins. (Pasteurizing became necessary because of the sanitation problems in dairies years ago. Today, these raw milk dairies are inspected frequently and have to meet a much higher standard than the dairies where milk is pasteurized.)

2) **Plenty of fresh vegetables and fruits, *not juiced,* but eaten in their whole form.** Vegetables and fruits need to be looked at for their carbohydrate content, which should be no more than 60 grams a day. (30 grams a day are recommended to lose weight, so you will need to purchase a carbohydrate and protein gram counter) Make sure that produce purchased is "certified organic". Again, in California, this means that farmers cannot use chemical fertilizers or pesticides for the previous 3 years. The soil is built up through organic means. After 3 years, the produce grown on this land is tested for pesticide residue. If there is none, then the label "certified organic" can be put on the produce, and in most cases this produce has **250%** more nutrients than commercially

grown produce. **If "certified organic" is not available, eat fresh produce anyway.**

3) **Water,** 6–8 glasses a day. (Avoid tap water, drink purified water instead.)

4) **Exercise.** You can't be optimally healthy just sitting or lying down all day long.

5) **1–3 tablespoons of raw olive oil every day—and use butter too.**

6) **Adequate amounts of all important vitamins and minerals taken daily, and whatever digestive enzymes you need. Remember, *supplements are the means of catching up for lost time nutritionally.* All of these should be determined by a health professional.**

How Does A Health Professional Know What You Need?

There are several methods used to determine the cause of your health problems. These techniques have all had successful results, and a health professional may use more than one. I have gone into detail only on those methods that most people are not familiar with:

1) **Blood, Saliva, Urine, and Hair Samples**

2) **Symptom Survey Forms**—These have been carefully worked out over a 10-year clinical trial period by many doctors. By using a grouping of symptoms, they can

help determine glandular imbalances, blood sugar handling, gall bladder function, etc…

3) **Reflex Analysis** — There are many reflex systems that have been developed over the last 70 years. Drs. DeJarnette, Rees, Barnett, Goodheart, and Versendaal have done extensive research on their reflex systems. Many trials matching blood and urine labwork have proved the accuracy of reflex analysis in determining the cause of any condition.

4) **Acoustic-Cardiograph Machine** — Based on the original phono-cardiograph invented by Dr. Lee, this machine has a microphone that "listens" to the heart beat and records the heart function graphically. An EKG machine measures an electrical current as it flows through the heart, and will only tell if damage or trauma has been done to the heart muscle. An Acoustic-Cardiograph can tell you if and where the heart is starting to malfunction. Any distortions in the beating pattern are picked up, recorded, and interpreted. It is important to note here that the heart *reflects the sum total of nutrition in the body.* The body will beg, borrow, and steal from its reserves to keep the heart healthy. If the heart is not functioning optimally, then what is getting put into the body is not doing the job. (Remember the sections on insulin and the damage it does.)

5) Clinical Experience — This is the overall picture of wellness the health professional gets by carefully observing his/her patient's skin tone, tongue, etc…

In summing up, I hope that the information in this booklet will set you firmly on the path to wellness. For further guidance, contact your health professional.

<u>Ode to a Shelf-Life</u>

Ah, but to last longer on the shelf
It certainly has made an industry of wealth

To enrich, store, and transport has been the goal
My body doesn't know the difference, I am told

If I could but last as long as thee
Oh odorless oils, canned foods, cereal, and
   candy

-Anonymous

If you like <u>Going Back to the Basics of Human Health</u>, be sure to read my next book, <u>The Biggest Cover-up of the 20th Century</u>..........You'll be amazed.

Footnotes

1. Jensen, Dr. Bernard and Mark Anderson, *Empty Harvest*, p. 14.
2. *Ibid*, p. 5.
3. *Ibid*, p. 73.
4. Liebig, Baron Justus von, *The Natural Laws of Husbandry.*
5. Jensen, Dr. Bernard and Mark Anderson, *Empty Harvest*, p. 75.
6. Howard, Sir Albert, *An Agricultural Testament*, Oxford University Press.
7. Jensen, Dr. Bernard and Mark Anderson, *Empty Harvest*, p. 32.
8. *Ibid*, pp. 57–58.
9. United States Deparment of Agriculture.
10. Jensen, Dr. Bernard and Mark Anderson, *Empty Harvest*, pp. 46–47.
11. *Ibid*, p. 8.
12. *Ibid*, p. 55.
13. *Ibid*, p. 7.
14. *Ibid*, p. 27.
15. *Ibid*.
16. *Ibid*, p. 97.
17. *Ibid*, p. 37.
18. Wiley, Dr. Harvey W., M.D., *The History of a Crime Against the Pure Food Law.*
19. *Washington Post*, October 26, 1949.
20. Jensen, Dr. Bernard and Mark Anderson, *Empty Harvest*, p. 36.
21. *bid*, p. 38.
22. *Ibid*.
23. *Ibid*.
24. *Ibid*, p. 39.
25. *Ibid*, p. 40.
26. *Ibid*, pp. 126-127.
27. West, B., M.D., "Oils and Disease", *Health Alert*, Vol. 11, Issue 3, (March 1994), p. 4; Dorman, Thomas A., M.D., *Search for Health*, (November 1994), p. 100.
28. DeCava, Judith A., M.S., LNC, *The Real Truth About Vitamins and Antioxidants*, p. 134.

29. *Ibid,* p. 140.
30. *Ibid.*
31. Jensen, Dr. Bernard and Mark Anderson, *Empty Harvest,* p. 136.
32. DeCava, Judith A., M.S., LNC, *The Real Truth About Vitamins and Antioxidants,* p. 76.
33. *Ibid,* p. 41–42.
34. Cheraskin, E. and W.M. Ringsdorf, Jr., *New Hope for Incurable Diseases,* (Jericho: Exposition, 1971), pp. 83–85.
35. DeCava, Judith A., M.S., LNC, *The Real Truth About Vitamins and Antioxidants,* p. 37.
36. Carter, Dr. James P., M.D., Dr.P.H., *Racketeering in Medicine,* pp. 23–24, citing David Horrobin, M.D., *Journal of the American Medical Association,* (March 1990), and Charles Harris, Pathologist, *Cult of Medical Science.*
37. Williams, Dr. Robert J., *Nutrition Against Disease,* pp. 4,5,11,17.
38. Krause, Marie V., B.S., M.S., R.D., and Kathleen Mahan, M.S., R.D., *Food, Nutrition and Diet Therapy,* (Philadelphia: W.B. Saunders Company, 1979), pp. 148–149.
39. DeCava, Judith A., M.S., LNC, *The Real Truth About Vitamins and Antioxidants,* p. 51.
40. *Ibid,* p. 57.
41. *Ibid.*
42. *Ibid,* p. 30.
43. *Ibid,* p. 31.
44. *Ibid,* p. 54.
45. *Ibid,* p. 128.
46. Levin, E., "Vitamin E vs. Wheat Germ Oil", *American Journal of Digestive Diseases,* Vol. 12, (January 1945), pp. 20–21.
47. *Scandinavian Veterinary,* Vol. 30, (1940), pp. 1121–1143, cited in *The Prevention Method for Better Health,* ed. J.I. Rodale, (Emmaus: Rodale Books, 1968), p. 568.
48. DeCava, Judith A., M.S., LNC, *The Real Truth About Vitamins and Antioxidants,* p. 190.

49. Jensen, Dr. Bernard and Mark Anderson, *Empty Harvest,* p. 123.
50. DeCava, Judith A., M.S., LNC, *The Real Truth About Vitamins and Antioxidants,* p. 41.
51. *Ibid,* p. 64.
52. Toufexis, Anastasia, *Time Magazine,* (6 April 1992), pp. 54–59.
53. DeCava, Judith A., M.S., LNC, *The Real Truth About Vitamins and Antioxidants,* p. 96.
54. *Ibid,* p. 70.
55. Challem, Jack, "Are You Overdoing Antioxidants?" *Natural Health,* Vol. 25, No. 3, (May/June 1995), pp. 56–57.
56. Jensen, Dr. Bernard and Mark Anderson, *Empty Harvest,* p. 25.
57. *Ibid,* p. 47.
58. *Ibid,* pp. 47–48.
59. Rodale, J.I., *The Complete Book of Food and Nutrition,* cited in *Empty Harvest,* pp. 127–128.
60. Eades, Michael R., M.D. and Mary Dan Eades, M.D., *Protein Power,* p. 25.
61. *Ibid,* p. 18.
62. *Ibid,* p. 25.
63. *Ibid,* p. 40.
64. Jensen, Arthur R., Ph.D., *Harvard Educational Review,* (Winter 1969) cited in *Protein Power,* p. 67.
65. Eades, Michael R., M.D. and Mary Dan Eades, M.D., *Protein Power,* pp. 50–51.
66. *Ibid,* pp. 113–114.
67. *Ibid,* p. 115.
68. *Ibid,* p. 117.
69. *Ibid,* p. 116.
70. *Ibid,* p. 51.
71. *Ibid,* p. 81.
72. *Ibid,* pp. 83–84.
73. *Ibid,* p. 110.
74. Atkins, Dr. Robert, *Health Revelations,* Vol. 4, No. 5, May 1996.

75. Willix, Robert D., Jr., M.D., *Maximum Health,* (Baltimore: Agora, Inc., 1993), pp. 33–35, cited in *The Real Truth About Vitamins and Antioxidants,* p. 35.
76. Jensen, Dr. Bernard and Mark Anderson, *Empty Harvest,* p.113.
77. Pottenger, Francis M., Jr., M.D., *Pottenger's Cats,* p. 93.
78. Davis, Adelle, M.S., *Let's Eat Right To Keep Fit,* p. 66.
79. Jensen, Dr. Bernard and Mark Anderson, *Empty Harvest,* pp. 153–154.
80. Murray, Richard P., D.C., P.A., *Natural vs. Synthetic Life vs. Death Truth vs. the Lie,* (1995), p. 4.
81. *ibid.*
82. *ibid,* p. 4–5.
83. DeCava, Judith A., M.S., LNC, *The Real Truth About Vitamins and Antioxidants,* p. 37.
84. DeCava, Judith A., M.S., LNC, *The Real Truth About Vitamins and Antioxidants,* p. 38.
85. West, Dr. Bruce, *Health Alert,* Vol. 14, No. 3, March 1997.
86. Eades, Michael R., M.D. and Mary Dan Eades, M.D., *Protein Power,* p. 114.
87. Eades, Michael R., M.D. and Mary Dan Eades, M.D., *Protein Power,* p. 137.

Suggested Reading:

1. *Empty Harvest,* Dr. Bernard Jensen and
   Mark Anderson
2. *The Real Truth About Vitamins and Antioxidants,*
   Judith A. DeCava, M.S., LNC
3. *Protein Power,* Michael R. Eades M.D. And
   Mary Dan Eades, M.D.
4. *Nutrition and Physical Degeneration,*
   Weston A. Price, D.D.S.
5. *Dr. Atkins' New Diet Revolution,*
   Robert C. Atkins, M.D.

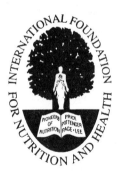

For more information
regarding the contents of
this book and the works of
the great pioneers in
nutrition, Drs. Royal Lee,
Melvin Page, Francis
Pottenger and Weston Price,
contact:

IFNH, 3963 Mission Blvd., San Diego, CA 92109
Ph: (619) 488-8932   Fax: (619) 488-2566

**Supporting the Healthcare Practitioner
through Seminars, Publications, and
Nutritional Evaluation Software**

ABOUT THE AUTHOR

Mary Frost is a nutritional journalist and researcher who has participated in the health field for over 25 years. She has uncovered many facts – some well-known, others buried in obscurity – which have made us rethink our knowledge and ideas of what good nutrition is.

Ms. Frost specializes in gathering nutritional information and putting the pieces together so the reader can comprehend the subject of nutrition and health in its entirety. Her particular focus is on foundational issues of health and nutrition and the negative impacts of today's lifestyle and diet. According to Ms. Frost, "I try to take the approach that a lot of people today are reading about nutrition and doctoring themselves. They are reading many books and trying to understand, but they find themselves more confused. In *Going Back to the Basics of Human Health*, I've tried to put it in easy-to-read language, summarizing it so people can quickly picture what truly makes them unhealthy. I want them to know how they got where they are."

Currently, Ms. Frost is working on another nutrition-oriented book that is yet to be titled. In it, she will investigate some of the greatest works ever done by the pioneers of nutrition such as Dr. Price's book titled *Nutrition and Physical Degeneration*, as well as Dr. Pottenger's book, *Pottenger's Cats*. In addition, Ms. Frost will summarize the body of work by Dr. Royal Lee, one of the 20th Century's true geniuses in clinical nutrition. Dr. Lee's depth of understanding of whole foods and the relationships of the vitamins and cofactors makes one wonder why we keep trying to reinvent the wheel.

An ongoing theme of Ms. Frost's new book will be how humankind regressed from looking at food as the basis of nutrition, to using synthesized chemicals and crystals and calling them nutrition. For instance, 90% of the Vitamin B sold in the United States is made from coal tar rather than food.

Ms. Frost herself encapsulated her next offering by stating, "I'm hoping to convey the biggest ongoing cover-up of the 20th and 21st Centuries. A lot of people are making quadrillions of dollars selling fake food and they don't want to be challenged. Health food stores are selling synthetic vitamins, puffed rice crackers that kill laboratory rats, and they don't even know it."